VIRUS REMEDIES GUIDEBOOK

Also by Deborah Bleecker

Acupuncture Points Handbook
Acupressure Made Simple
Tung Acupuncture Points
Acupuncture for Migraines
Shingles Relief
Natural Back Pain Solutions
Insomnia Relief

VIRUS REMEDIES GUIDEBOOK

A Practical Guide
to the Most Effective Virus Remedies,
and How to Use Them to
Help Yourself

Deborah Bleecker, LAc, MSOM

Disclaimer

This book contains the opinions and ideas of the author. It is intended to provide helpful and informative material on the subject addressed. It is sold with the understanding that the author and publisher are not engaged in rendering medical, health, psychological or any other type of advice or services in the book. If the reader needs personal, medical, health, or other assistance or advice, a competent professional should be consulted.

The author and publisher disclaim any responsibility for any liability, loss or risk, either personal or otherwise that occurs as a consequence, directly or indirectly, of the use and application of the contents of this book.

Draycott Publishing, LLC

ISBN: 978-1-940146-96-6
Library of Congress Control Number: 2021922354

Contents

Introduction

This book is a compilation of everything I believe you need to know about treating viral infections with natural medicine. I have a Master of Science degree in Oriental Medicine, which is a three-year program of study on how to treat disease with acupuncture and Chinese herbal medicine. I have been treating colds and flu with herbs for over 24 years.

The products presented in this book are available over the counter. They are easy to buy, and easy to use. I give you the same information I have given my patients for years on how to treat viral infections quickly and effectively.

There Are Possibly Hundreds of Antiviral Herbs

There are dozens of herbs used in Traditional Chinese Medicine, abbreviated as TCM. These herbs have been used for thousands of years. They have a history of safe and effective usage. There are also dozens if not hundreds of effective antiviral herbs that have been used in many countries.

I Am Not Making This Stuff Up

One of the arguments that is often made against herbal medicine is that although the herbs have a long history of usage, they have not been proven to be effective. They argue that it is "all anecdotal." This is why I have done extensive research that confirms the usage of the herbs and vitamins I include in this book.

The research HAS been done already. Research on using natural medicine to treat viral infections has been done for many years. The pace of research has accelerated since the COVID-19 pandemic started.

I think it is important to make the research easy to find. So, I have included the references within the section on each supplement. There is already so much research on these antiviral herbs, that I had to choose one or two that stood out, and include those references.

Some of the most powerful antiviral herbs are those used in Chinese medicine. There are also many herbs used in America, and the West, which are very effective antivirals. Although my experience using Chinese herbs to treat viruses is more extensive.

First, Do No Harm

The herbal medicines and other supplements in this book have been used for hundreds, if not thousands of years. I usually tell my patients that most herbs are so safe, that you could even take the whole bottle at once, and your only side effect might be temporary intestinal problems.

The annual cost to prevent a cold or flu from becoming a serious illness could be as little as $30. If herbs and vitamins are taken early and often, it is often easy to knock out a virus in a day or two. That said, all information in this book is for educational purposes only. Always consult your medical doctor.

Treat Early and Often, and As Long as You Need

You will get sick of reading it, but I will say it over and over again that you should treat any infection as soon as you can, and keep treating it. There is really no downside to these remedies that would ever outweigh the possible residual effects of viruses. Even if you think you are already over a virus, you could consider taking a course of the antivirals in this book. Viral infections often linger, even if you have no symptoms.

Although it is best to treat infections early, it is never too late.

Viral Stage
Does Not Matter

Antiviral supplements can be taken at any stage of an infection.

Up to 650,000 People Annually

As of 2017, the average death toll worldwide for colds and flu, and all the associated ailments such as bronchitis, and pneumonia, is up to 650,000. Most people do not know how deadly the average flu virus can be, and how important it is to treat it effectively.

It is up to You to Protect Yourself

Only you can decide if you want to try safe and simple remedies. I understand that a lot of people will simply not believe it if someone says that herbs can be used as antivirals, even with modern research confirming it. But what is the downside?

I always recommend to my patients and family to keep antiviral herbs available at all times. If you think you have a virus, or have been exposed to one, there is little reason not to take the herbs to treat it quickly.

Practical Guide

My goal with this book is not to give you a huge list of obscure herbs or supplements. It is important to me that you are able to find and use the supplements easily. I have included the brands I have personally tested, as well as the dosage I would personally take. I do not receive any compensation for the supplements I recommend.

Chinese Herb Names

I am including the name of the Chinese herbs in this book so you can easily do more research online, if you are interested. If you look for the common name, or the Latin name, it is harder to find the correct herb.

1

How to Choose Effective Herbal Medicines

It can be tricky to choose quality herbal medicines. That is why I usually include my top choices for brands and products. I am not affiliated with these companies and am not compensated in any way. I remember what it is like to feel overwhelmed when trying to buy supplements. Some products are not very effective, and you can waste your money and your time on them.

Herbal Extracts

There are two basic types of herb products. One is a bulk herb, where the herb is just ground up and encapsulated. The other is an extract. An extract is made by boiling the herb in water for twenty to thirty minutes. The liquid from this is dehydrated, which leaves behind a strong herbal extract powder, with the fiber essentially removed.

An Herbal Extract is Easier to Digest

Most herbs are roots. That means they are not easy to digest. You might get some benefit, but herbal extracts are easier to digest, and much stronger.

Some herbs are easier to digest. An example of this would be gotu kola. This is a leaf, and it is easy to digest. Herbs like astragalus root are a woody root, and should be taken as an extract. If I have a choice, I always choose an extract.

Take Fewer Pills with An Extract

If you use raw herbal powders, you will need to take at least three or four times as many pills as you would have to take with an extract. If an extract is 4 x, that means that the one tablet of the extract is the extraction of four times the amount of herb.

There is currently no standardized extraction guideline. The definition of 4x could be seen as four times as strong as the raw root, but there is no rule to apply to this definition. Taking herbs from a reputable company is important.

An Extract Does Not Have to Be a Liquid

The term “herbal extract” does not mean the herb is in liquid form. You can buy an extracted herb in a tablet, capsule, powder, or a liquid. The herbs are still usually extracted with water, and preserved with alcohol. Some herbs are extracted with alcohol, but this is not as common.

Herb Standardization

An herb that is “standardized” means that it has been tested to verify that is has a certain level of a specific compound. When an herb is standardized, this does not mean that the standardized component is the most important part of the herb.

Standardization is just used as a means of measuring the potency, and quality of the herb. It is usually best if you can buy an herb that has been standardized. Pharmaceutical grade Chinese herbs are not standardized, because the process of making them involves checking each herb in a lab to ensure it is the correct herb, and that it contains what it is supposed to contain.

If you buy herbs from established herb companies, you can generally trust they have done their research, and had the herbs tested for quality and potency before they sell them.

Herbal Compounds, or Components

Each herb might have dozens or hundreds of compounds. Researchers will sometimes extract what they believe to be the most important active compound in an herb. They choose to research isolated compounds, rather than the complete herb.

Taking herbs in their original, and complete form is how you benefit from the safety of herbal medicine. One isolated compound, taken alone, might cause side effects.

When someone uses only the isolated compound from an herb, not the whole herb, it is basically a drug, in my opinion.

Whole herbs have been used for thousands of years, so they cannot be patented. There is not a lot of money to be made in selling herbal supplements, compared to selling pharmaceuticals. That is why a lot of research is done using isolated compounds, since those products can be patented.

Be Careful of Excipients

An excipient is something added to bulk up the herb to make it easier to make into tablets, or into capsules. When you look at the label of a supplement, you want to make sure how much of the active ingredient you are getting per capsule.

Some companies add corn starch, or rice to stretch the herbs. I have also seen companies add oil. In trying to find a green powder supplement such as a combination of barley grass juice, wheat grass juice, and other juice extracts, you will often see fiber added to stretch it. Oat fiber and flax fiber are added to bulk the product up. Some companies add extra oil such as sunflower oil, to stretch the ingredients.

Not all excipients are bad, or made to stretch the product. Sometimes manufacturers have to add something to make the product into tablets. Also, sometimes fiber is wanted in the product. Just be sure to compare products with that in mind.

Herbal Teas

Herbal teas should be brewed for 15 to 20 minutes. Regular tea is usually brewed for three to five minutes. But to get the full benefit of herbal tea, they need more time to brew properly.

2

Why You Should Use Herbal Medicine to Protect Yourself

The following is my opinion, based on my research.

Viruses Mutate Constantly

Viruses mutate. It is virtually the defining characteristic of viruses that they mutate. They change their tactics based on how to enhance their own survival. If they kill a host too fast, they will not be able to spread their DNA and survive long term. The host will be dead, and no longer able to spread the virus.

Their goal is to spread to as many people as possible, for their own survival. Although it is said that viruses are not alive, they are just bits of DNA, I have not figured out how something that is not alive can mutate, so for the purposes of this book, I consider them to be alive. I guess it depends on what your definition of alive is.

Viruses are Tiny

Some people say that viruses can easily pass through the holes in some face masks. The tiny holes in some face masks are much larger than the viral particles. In addition, the viral particles can also enter around the edges of masks. Viruses can be transferred to your eyes from your hands very easily. Once they contact a mucus membrane, they can spread all over your body. It is not possible to be completely protected from infections.

You Often Do Not Know You Were Exposed to a Virus

Unless you have obvious symptoms, you might not know you have been exposed to a virus. You would need to know the symptoms of the virus, and there are thousands of viruses.

You are exposed to viruses all the time, and will not even know it unless your immune system is low, and the virus is able to overcome your natural immune system protection.

Viruses Are Everywhere, You Cannot Avoid Them

Viral particles are left on surfaces, like shopping carts, counter tops, pens, keyboards, and light switches. It is almost impossible to not be exposed to many different types of viruses every day. It can make you paranoid if you think about it.

What is Immunity?

Bear with me on this one. I believe that even if you have been exposed to a virus, and recovered from it, you are not necessarily fully protected forever. If your immune system becomes weak, you might catch that virus again.

Immunity means your body recognizes the virus. It has already made antibodies to it, so it will respond faster. But what if the virus has already mutated? This is a big question, and I think it is hard to know for sure. I am not a virus expert.

It is possible to take herbs that kill viruses directly, stop the virus from attaching to your own cells and reproducing, as well as boost your immune system, so your body can protect you from it.

A healthy immune system is the key to surviving viruses. Your immune system is the only thing keeping you alive. If it is strong, and you are generally healthy, you are much less likely to get horribly sick. However, it is easy to get run down, and not even realize it.

Some Viruses Stay in Your Body Forever

Viruses like Hepatitis stay in your body forever. There is no way to confirm that you have actually gotten rid of a virus. It might not be possible. The symptoms might be gone, but is the virus gone?

You will never completely kill all viruses in your body. Many viruses are actually useful to us and work with us. Your immune system needs to work in order to identify and destroy the viruses that are harmful to us.

320,000 Different Viruses Infect Mammals

It is not possible to know exactly how many viruses there are in existence. They are everywhere. Viruses like Epstein Barr and

Chickenpox, for example, are believed to never really leave the body.

Chickenpox is believed to hide in your body and when your immune system is low, due to stress, or fatigue, it can attack your spinal nerves and cause shingles. This is a horrible disease, and if you are armed with the right supplements, you might be able to prevent its progression. The earlier you treat any virus, the better your results will be.

3

Is It a Virus? How To Catch A Virus In The Early Stages

Colds and flu and other viruses can sneak up on you. Since it is much easier to resolve viruses if you catch them early, you need to be able to recognize the virus symptoms as soon as possible.

The longer a virus is in your body, the more it is able to make more copies of itself. A virus replicating is taking over your cells and building up an army against you. The sooner you start your defense and offense, the sooner you can recover.

I am Repeating This on Purpose

The sooner you treat a virus, the better your results. Don't wait until you have horrible symptoms. Natural medicine is very safe, and it makes no sense to wait.

Chinese Medicine Theory Makes It Clear

Since Chinese herbal medicine has been used to treat viruses and epidemic diseases for thousands of years, the symptoms of each phase of infection have been systematized.

Chinese medicine theory stages can tell you how far along your infection is. The sooner you can take herbs in the clear heat toxin category, the faster you will recover. The virus will not have time to reproduce itself and build up an army against your immune system.

Please note that some viruses have different symptoms in the early stages, and throughout. However, these guidelines will help.

Antiviral Herbs Treat Any Stage

The treatment in the early stages is the same for any virus. It can also be difficult to distinguish between allergies, and cold or flu. However, the herbs used in Chinese medicine will help to destroy viruses at any stage, so there is no need to worry. Take the supplements explained in this book early and often.

DO not wait! Take herbs and supplements at the first sign of a virus, as well as when you might have been exposed to one. In my experience, if you catch the virus and take herbs in the first day or two, you might only need to take the supplements once or twice. It depends on the virus and the health of your immune system. Your immune system keeps you alive.

Chinese Medicine Made Simple

The following information is very basic. I have not included the later stages of infection, because they vary, and your herbal choices do not need to change.

An acupuncturist will look at your tongue, and take your pulse, but that information is not relevant to someone who does not have experience making a diagnosis. It takes training and experience to differentiate tongue colors and the quality of pulses. This information is not necessary to treat viruses in the early stages.

Wind Cold Symptoms – The First Stage

The first stage of a viral infection. At this stage, you might not know you have been exposed to a virus. You might feel chills, have a slight runny nose, sneeze a little, or have a headache. If you can get used to spotting these symptoms, you will get great results treating viruses.

Although you only need to have ONE of these symptoms to suspect you might have been exposed to a virus, the symptoms are:

- Aversion to cold
- Coughing

- No fever, or slight fever
- No sweating
- No thirst
- Runny nose with clear or white mucus
- Sneezing
- Tight neck muscles at base of skull

Wind Heat Symptoms – Second Stage

This is the stage where most people notice something is going on. You might have a fever, and the virus is starting to cause more severe symptoms. You might feel a sore throat, feel chills, or the start of a fever.

- Aversion to cold
- Cough
- Fever
- Itchy or sore throat
- Runny nose with yellow mucus
- Shivering
- Sneezing
- Swollen tonsils
- Thirst
- Tight neck muscles at base of skull

Phlegm Heat – It Is Getting Serious

In advanced stages of viral infection, your body produces a lot of yellow phlegm or mucus. You might also have a dry mouth and lips, and no mucus.

There are herbs that treat the mucus aspect of this phase, but in my experience, it is best to focus on killing the virus, since the mucus is being produced by your body to protect you from being damaged by the virus. If you kill the virus and boost your immune system, the mucus often takes care of itself.

If the mucus is copious, herbal cough syrups can be used to dissolve the mucus, and relieve coughing, while you continue with antiviral supplements.

Mucus Is There to Protect You

If you are coughing mucus, it is possible that bacteria have already started accumulating in your lungs. If you take drugs or even herbs to stop the mucus production, or to dissolve it, you can dry up the mucus and make the viral infection much worse. It is always best to focus on treating the virus, and boosting the immune system.

If you are already treating the virus, and are still coughing mucus, there are herbal cough remedies in Chinese medicine that are used to resolve the mucus and stop coughing. An example of this type of formula is Loquat Respiratory Syrup from Planetary Herbals.

The herbs in this cough syrup are listed as: Loquat Leaf, Zhejiang Fritillary Bulb, Black Cherry Bark, Slippery Elm Bark, Platycodon Root, Trichosanthes Seed, Polygala Root, Poria Sclerotium, Schisandra Fruit, Chinese Licorice Root and Rhizome.

Loquat leaf is called Pi Pa Ye in Chinese. It is used for coughing and wheezing. It resolves mucus, clears lung inflammation, restores normal lung function, and relieves coughing. It also helps to regulate the stomach.

Fritillary is called Zhe Bei Mu in Chinese. It is used to treat mucus, and inflammation, and relieve a productive cough. It is also used for nodules in the neck, lung and breast abscesses, and swellings.

Platycodon root is called Jie Geng in Chinese. It treats mucus, it regulates the lungs, expels mucus. It also treats sore throat.

Trichosanthes seed is called Gua Lou Ren. It is the seeds of the trichosanthes. Three parts of this herb are used to treat the lungs, the fruit, seeds, and root. They have different functions.

Trichosanthes seeds clear and transform inflammation and mucus. It treats cough with chest pain.

Polygala is called Yuan Zhi in Chinese. It is in the heart calming category of herbs. It also expels phlegm from the lungs. It treats coughs with copious sputum, especially when difficult to expectorate.

Poria is called Fu Ling in Chinese. Poria strengthens digestion, and helps to resolve mucus.

Schisandra fruit is called Wu Wei Zi. It is used to strengthen the lungs to relieve coughing. This herb has a lot of additional functions, but that is what it is used for in this formula.

Chinese licorice root is called Gan Cao. Licorice root strengthens digestion, moistens the lungs, and stops coughing, as used in this formula. It also has many uses.

Most of the herbs in this formula have been used by herbalists for years to resolve coughs with mucus production. It should not be used for a dry cough. I have used a cough syrup formula similar to this for years. It can often quickly resolve coughing. Some of the herbs are to resolve the mucus, and some stop coughing. Black cherry bark, and other herbs not explained here are used in Western herbal medicine. The Chinese formula was modified with Western herbs.

Lung Energy Weakness after a Cold or Flu is over

If you have recovered from a cold or flu, but you are still coughing and feel weak, you might have a residual viral or bacterial infection, or you could be weak after fighting off the infection. The cough is usually a weak cough.

You have to analyze the cough. A weak cough, vs. a deep cough are caused by different things. A deep cough is usually caused by mucus remaining in the lungs. Your lungs could be inflamed, but you definitely need to get medical help for that.

If the mucus remains in your lungs, it can easily harbor bacteria, which can block your lungs and kill you!

Breathing Problems

If you have any breathing problems whatsoever, you need to seek medical help. It is not uncommon to get a bacterial infection in your lungs. In addition to the fact that viruses like COVID-19 attack your lungs directly.

Treating a cold or flu when the first symptoms appear will make an upper respiratory infection, bronchitis, or pneumonia a lot less likely to occur.

Always See a Medical Doctor for Lung Symptoms

Any lung symptom, chest tightness, coughing mucus, or difficulty breathing is very serious.

Although I avoid taking pharmaceuticals, I would not hesitate to take antibiotics for any type of lung infection.

When you are infected, your body expends a lot of energy to battle the virus. This combined with coughing and the virus possibly attacking your lungs directly, will weaken your lungs and cause you to have symptoms for a long time. Please refer to the chapter on Colds and Flu Recovery for more information on residual flu symptoms.

Spanish Flu Pandemic of 1918

There are many types of viruses, and each one will have possible symptoms. To illustrate this, I have included information on the Spanish Flu.

Notice that it says the majority of deaths were caused by bacterial pneumonia. Most herbs that treat viruses also treat bacteria, and if necessary, most of them can be taken for months if needed, to make sure the body has fully recovered.

The following information is an excerpt from Wikipedia information on the Spanish Flu:

"The majority of the infected experienced only the typical flu symptoms of sore throat, headache, and fever, especially during the first wave. However, during the second wave, the disease was much more serious, often complicated by bacterial pneumonia, which was often the cause of death. This more serious type would cause *heliotrope cyanosis* to develop, whereby the skin would first develop two mahogany spots over the cheekbones which would then over a few hours spread to color the entire face blue, followed by black coloration first in the extremities and then further spreading to the limbs and the torso. After this, death would follow within hours or days due to the lungs being filled with fluids.

Other signs and symptoms reported included spontaneous mouth and nosebleeds, miscarriages for pregnant women, a peculiar smell, teeth, and hair falling, delirium, dizziness, insomnia, loss of hearing or smell, blurred vision, and impaired color vision. One observer wrote, "One of the most striking of the complications was hemorrhage from mucous membranes, especially from the nose, stomach, and intestine. Bleeding from the ears and petechial hemorrhages in the skin also occurred". The severity of the symptoms was believed to be caused by cytokine storms.

The majority of deaths were from bacterial pneumonia, a common secondary infection associated with influenza. This pneumonia was itself caused by common upper respiratory-tract bacteria, which were able to get into the lungs via the damaged bronchial tubes of the victims.

The virus also killed people directly by causing massive hemorrhages and edema in the lungs. Modern analysis has shown the virus to be particularly deadly because it triggers a cytokine storm (overreaction of the body's immune system). One group of researchers recovered the virus from the bodies of frozen victims and transfected animals with it. The animals suffered rapidly progressive respiratory failure and death through a cytokine storm. The strong immune reactions of young adults were postulated to have ravaged the body, whereas the weaker immune reactions of children and middle-aged adults resulted in fewer deaths among those groups."

Please bear in mind that viral infections can easily lead to bacterial infections. The infection might start with a virus, but if the immune system is impaired, bacteria can build up as a secondary infection. The herbs that kill viruses, also usually kill bacteria.

Herbs that treat <u>viruses</u>
are usually also
effective against
<u>bacteria</u>

Notice how the Spanish flu symptoms included bleeding. In Chinese medicine theory, symptoms such as purple lips, purple spots on the body, nosebleeds, hemorrhage, bleeding from the ears would be treated with herbs that cool and thin the blood.

Curcumin is an herb in that category, but it is a relatively mild one. Please refer to the chapter on blood clot prevention and treatment.

Chronic Viral Infections

There are many types of viruses, the type that cause the common cold or flu are easily recognizable from the symptoms listed above. Other viruses are harder to spot, and the only symptom might be fatigue. These types of viruses can linger in the body and cause chronic fatigue symptoms. Some people are tired all the time, and they do not know that a virus is the cause of their fatigue.

The virus remedies in this book can be used to treat any type of virus. The mechanism is the same. Attack the virus directly, and boost your immune system. If you have lingering fatigue and have been able to rule out other causes, taking antiviral supplements for a while might help you.

These supplements are usually effective against bacteria, as well as fungi such as Candida. All these pathogens wear you down, because your body has to focus on killing the virus infected cells, rather than giving you extra energy to focus on your day. Your body is fighting for its life, and fatigue is a side effect.

COVID-19 Symptoms

Although COVID-19 is still evolving, and we are learning more every day, it might be helpful to include information on some of the symptoms here.

The COVID-19 virus has unusual symptoms. Here I am quoting the Centers for Disease Control, at CDC.gov:

"People with COVID-19 have had a wide range of symptoms reported – ranging from mild symptoms to severe illness. Symptoms may appear 2-14 days after exposure to the virus. Anyone can have mild to severe symptoms. People with these symptoms may have COVID-19:

- Fever or chills
- Cough
- Shortness of breath or difficulty breathing
- Fatigue
- Muscle or body aches
- Headache

- New loss of taste or smell
- Sore throat
- Congestion or runny nose
- Nausea or vomiting
- Diarrhea

This list does not include all possible symptoms. CDC will continue to update this list as we learn more about COVID-19. Older adults and people who have severe underlying medical conditions like heart or lung disease or diabetes seem to be at higher risk for developing more serious complications from COVID-19 illness."

"Look for emergency warning signs* for COVID-19. If someone is showing any of these signs, **seek emergency medical care immediately:**

- Trouble breathing
- Persistent pain or pressure in the chest
- New confusion
- Inability to wake or stay awake
- Pale, gray, or blue-colored skin, lips, or nail beds, depending on skin tone

*This list is not all possible symptoms. Please call your medical provider for any other symptoms that are severe or concerning to you."

Unusual COVID-19 Symptoms

There are a few symptoms that are not commonly published. I do believe that this list will grow over time.

- Whole-body rashes
- Swelling and redness in just a few spots
- Loss of appetite
- Pinkeye
- Abdominal pain

COVID-19 Can Attack Organs

Research is still being done on how Covid attacks the organs. Since this is a new virus, more information on how and what it attacks will be available as time goes on.

COVID-19 has been known to damage the lungs, kidneys, heart, liver, central nervous system, blood vessels, and the intestines.

Is it a Heart Attack or COVID-19?

I personally had strong palpitations and racing heart for several days. I finally realized that it might be COVID-19, so I took antiviral herbs for a few days and the heart symptoms stopped. One of my neighbors called an ambulance thinking she was having a heart attack. It was COVID-19.

If I had not had antiviral herbs available, I might have succumbed to those heart symptoms. The virus is attacking the heart muscle and damaging it. Palpitations and heart symptoms are always serious, always seek medical help.

Sense of Smell, and Taste with COVID-19

I think one of the most common symptoms of this virus is the loss of the sense of smell and taste. Some people are not recovering their sense of smell after they get over the virus. It is not known if this is permanent damage to the nerve that is responsible for smell, or a lingering virus. If I had a lingering lack of taste and smell, I would assume I might have a virus lingering also, and treat it with antivirals.

At this point, if I had any weird symptom at all, during the COVID-19 pandemic, I would personally take supplements to treat viruses.

If the problem with the lack of ability to smell and taste still persisted, I would get acupuncture on Large Intestine 20, which is right by the nose. This point "opens the nose" which helps you to smell better. I believe it probably stimulates the nerves in the nose to improve their function. I have written an acupuncture point book for patients called *Acupuncture Points Handbook*, which goes over the points in detail.

Acupressure For Loss of Smell Sensation

For loss of, or reduction in the ability to smell, you could try acupressure. If you press firmly, you will probably feel a tenderness. Press each side for five minutes, and repeat if necessary. You can treat these points as many times as you want.

The image below is of Large Intestine 20. This point might be enough to restore your sense of smell, if you use it daily for a few weeks. I would treat it twice a day, five minutes per side. There is no harm in doing it more often. Press as firmly as possible to stimulate the nerve. If this does not work, I would get acupuncture, which is a stronger stimulation of the nerves. It is more likely to work

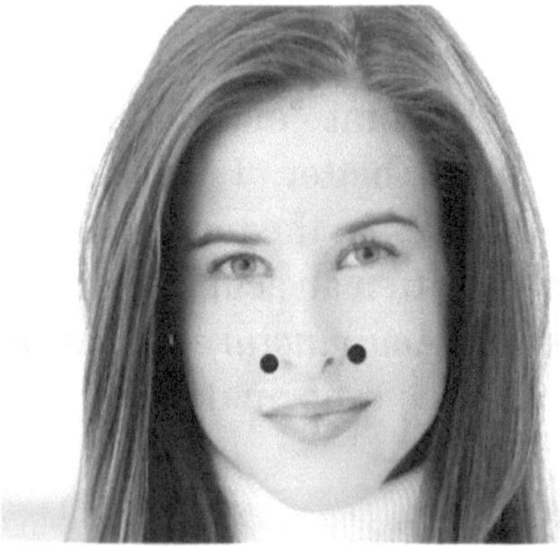

Acupressure Point for
Sense of Smell

than acupressure.

The image below shows the olfactory nerve. This is what they believe is affected by the virus, which causes the problems with smelling and tasting. As you can see from the location of the nerve, anything in the sinuses can affect it.

I once had a patient who could not smell at all. His daughter was upset, because she was afraid that he would accidentally eat spoiled food, not knowing it was off. I treated him for sinus infection and inflammation, and we were able to restore his sense of smell.

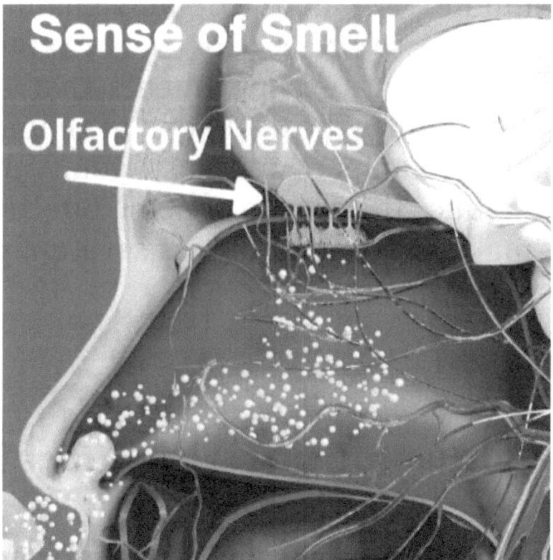

Treat any infection early and often

We do not know how long COVID-19 and the variants it creates will be around. Viruses always mutate. We have to be vigilant about symptoms. Please refer to the chapter on prevention. There are supplements that can be taken daily to reduce the likelihood of an infection. Herbs and vitamins can boost your immune system to reduce the chance of being infected, and possibly make the symptoms less severe if you do get infected.

Stealth Viruses, Do You Have One?

Fatigue is a common problem, and it is diagnosed and treated in Chinese medicine. It is fairly easy to treat fatigue with herbal medicine and acupuncture. However, a few years ago I had a patient who taught me a lesson.

Sarah was in her 70's. She was referred to me because she had crushing fatigue. She said she could not get out of bed. She wanted to sleep all the time. She was usually very active in her church, and she was not the type of person to nap regularly.

I thought it would be pretty simple to treat her fatigue. There are dozens of herbal formulas used to treat fatigue. Acupuncturists treat fatigue all the time, it is an important part of our job as acupuncturists.

I treated her with acupuncture and Chinese herbs for a few weeks. She was getting better, a little bit at a time. However, after a couple of weeks of treating her, I personally started wanting to sleep all day. I could not pass by my bed without wanting to climb in it and just lie there. That is not normal for me either.

Then it hit me. She had a virus! Her fatigue was caused by some type of virus, and she had passed it on to me. I had the exact same symptoms as she did. The main symptom was fatigue, but in addition to that, one eye watered regularly, for no apparent reason.

There is no way to know what virus it was. We are all a pea soup of the viruses we are exposed to. If we are strong enough, we knock the virus out and it does not get a chance to take over. In my case, I had recently moved, so my body had gone through a lot, and I was not well enough to fight off the virus quickly.

Since this was not a respiratory virus, like a cold or flu, I was not sure if the herbs I normally used for that were appropriate. I now know that they would have been great to treat any type of virus.

I chose olive leaf extract. I knew it was effective as a broad-spectrum antiviral. I learned that I needed to take 1,000 mg. two to three times a day for several weeks. If I did not do that, the virus would come back, and I would be tired all day, with the one eye watering on and off all day.

This incident was several years ago, before I knew about vitamin C being such a strong antiviral. I would have included 10,000 to 15,000 mg daily in powder form if I had known then what I know now.

Sarah has taken different ginseng formulations, and kidney tonics, in addition to the antivirals, and she is now thriving.

Blood Sugar Levels and Viruses

There is evidence that insulin resistance and high blood sugar levels are associated with not being able to fight off viruses. Sugar also competes with vitamin C for absorption, so you will not absorb your vitamin C as well if you take it with sugar. Lower carbohydrate intake might improve your ability to fight off viruses.

4

Antiviral Herbal Medicine, Single Herbs, Western

There are hundreds of herbs that can be used as antivirals. I am including in this chapter only the ones I believe are the most dependable. I have excluded things that are not traditionally used as antivirals, if I believe they are not dependable for that.

I'm Still Not Making This Stuff Up

As I mentioned at the beginning of this book, although many of these herbs have been used for hundreds if not thousands of years to treat the symptoms of viral infections, I feel it is important to include modern research confirming their usage.

There are hundreds of studies available, with more research being done all the time. If you would like to verify these research articles, you can simply search online for the name of the study, and PubMed, which is the US government website for scientific research. The research details are included after the herb or supplement, for easy confirmation.

Olive Leaf Extract

This is one of my favorite Western herbs to treat viruses. It is derived from olive leaves, but interestingly it is also present in olive oil in smaller amounts. Olive leaf kills viruses, bacteria, and fungi.

Olive leaf is typically sold as a standardized extract. Always check the smell of this herb. If it smells strong, it is usually a good indicator of a quality product.

Nature's Way makes a standardized extract product. Each capsule has 250 mg. of 12% oleuropein. Planetary Herbals makes a product with each tablet containing 700 mg. olive leaf extract, standardized at 10% oleuropein. I typically recommend 500 mg. minimum per dosage, three to four times a day.

In addition to taking this internally, olive leaf extract has been shown to be effective against viruses topically.

Research:

Alhadrami HA, Sayed AM, Sharif AM, Azhar EI, Rateb ME. Olive-Derived Triterpenes Suppress SARS COV-2 Main Protease: A Promising Scaffold for Future Therapeutics. Molecules. 2021 May 1;26(9):2654. doi:

10.3390/molecules26092654. PMID: 34062737; PMCID: PMC8125615.

Oregano Oil and Thyme

Oregano oil is traditionally used most often to treat Candida and other fungal infections. It can be taken internally, and the oil can be applied topically. It contains a compound called carvacrol, which is reported to be anti-cancer, anti-fungal, anti-bacterial, anti-oxidant, anti-inflammatory, and it has liver protective effects. These herbs affect the ability of the virus to attach to the cell and start reproducing. This is the most common modern description of how most antiviral herbs work. Black cumin seed also has carvacrol.

I personally like the Nature's Way brand, which has 75-85% carvacrol, with 50 mg. per capsule. This is very strong, and I would suggest taking a low dose. More is not necessarily better with this one. In the case of oregano oil and thyme, I believe a standardized product is important.

Since oregano oil also kills the Candida intestinal fungus, you might get a die off reaction if you take too much at one time.

Research:

Javed H, Meeran MFN, Jha NK, Ojha S. Carvacrol, a Plant Metabolite Targeting Viral Protease (M^{pro}) and ACE2 in Host Cells Can Be a Possible Candidate for COVID-19. Front Plant Sci. 2021 Feb 16;11:601335. doi: 10.3389/fpls.2020.601335. PMID: 33664752; PMCID: PMC7921315.

Research:

Swamy MK, Akhtar MS, Sinniah UR. Antimicrobial Properties of Plant Essential Oils against Human Pathogens and Their Mode of Action: An Updated Review. Evid Based Complement Alternat Med. 2016;2016:3012462. doi: 10.1155/2016/3012462. Epub 2016 Dec 20. PMID: 28090211; PMCID: PMC5206475.

Holy Basil, Tulsi

Holy basil is an herb commonly used in Ayurvedic herbal medicine, originating in India. I do not have personal experience of using this herb against viruses, but it was mentioned so often in research studies, that I wanted to include it.

Holy basil is not like common basil, used for cooking. It is used to treat stress, anxiety, and is an antidepressant. Keep in mind that depression always has a cause. Depression can be caused by Candida, food allergies, and omega 3 oil deficiencies. Chronic high levels of inflammation can also affect the brain. These are possible reasons why holy basil might help treat depression.

Holy basil also treats bacteria, viruses, fungi, and is a natural anti-inflammatory. It also contains the compound carvacrol, as does oregano oil and thyme.

The following report discusses numerous Indian herbs that might be helpful against viruses.

Research:

Gautam S, Gautam A, Chhetri S, Bhattarai U. Immunity Against COVID-19: Potential Role of Ayush Kwath. J Ayurveda Integr Med. 2020 Aug 17. doi: 10.1016/j.jaim.2020.08.003. Epub ahead of print. PMID: 32837101; PMCID: PMC7430223.

Elderberry

I am only including elderberry in this book, because so many people try it as an antiviral. I would not depend on it. I have personally not had good results when I tried it. There might be several reasons why.

Elderberry liquid often includes a lot of sugar. Sugar suppresses the immune system. It also competes with vitamin C for absorption. If you take vitamin C when you have high blood sugar, you will absorb less vitamin C.

Elderberry is usually taken as a liquid. So, the high amount of water dilutes the amount of the active herb. So perhaps capsules would be more effective. I cannot recommend this herb, especially during a time that we are currently going through a pandemic. You cannot take chances.

The research I found on elderberry was very weak. If you have taken this herb in the past and had success with it, you might find even better results with some of the other herbs in this book. I suspect you would recover faster by taking andrographis, or other herbs.

Stephen Harrod Buhner, in his book, *Herbal Antivirals, 2nd Edition*, states that in his opinion elderberry is a narrow spectrum antiviral. He says he suspects it is because the elder leaves and bark are stronger than the berries, but rarely used. He writes "If you have nothing else handy for a severe respiratory infection, use it." I could not agree more.

Research:

1. Zakay-Rones Z, Thom E, Wollan T, Wadstein J. Randomized Study of the Efficacy and Safety of Oral Elderberry Extract in the Treatment of Influenza A and B Virus Infections. Journal of International Medical Research. April 2004:132-140. doi:10.1177/147323000403200205

Echinacea

Echinacea is typically used to improve the immune system, to help the body resolve viral infections. It can be helpful, but I would personally not choose this herb. My first choice would always be the Chinese herbs, explained in other chapters, but in case they are not available, echinacea is an option.

Echinacea is effective for a few weeks at a time to boost the immune system. It is not effective if taken long term. It stops working, after about three weeks. There are different types of immune tonic herbs. Deep immune tonics like astragalus will continue to strengthen your immune system. Echinacea is not a deep tonic. It should be taken as a liquid extract only. The pills are just not strong enough to treat a serious infection.

I did get good results with echinacea once, when I did not have access to Chinese herbs. I gave the person echinacea liquid every hour or two, and I also did acupuncture several times a day.

My book, *Acupressure Made Simple*, explains how to use acupressure points to treat colds and flu. Stomach 36, and 40 are used to boost the immune system and resolve the infection. Large Intestine 4, and 11 strengthen the immune system, and clear fever.

Echinacea extract brands I would try, in order of preference are: A. Vogel Echinaforce, Planetary Herbals, Herb Pharm, NOW, Nature's Way, Gaia, and Pure Mountain Botanicals. All of these brands make a liquid extract.

The research I found on echinacea indicates that "the results were consistent with a decrease in the pro-inflammatory cytokines that play a role in the progression of cytokine storm and Acute Respiratory Distress Syndrome (ARDS), factors that play a significant role in the death of COVID-19 patients."

Research:

Aucoin M, Cooley K, Saunders PR, Carè J, Anheyer D, Medina DN, Cardozo V, Remy D, Hannan N, Garber A. The effect of *Echinacea* spp. on the prevention or treatment of COVID-19 and other respiratory tract infections in humans: A rapid review. Adv Integr Med. 2020 Dec;7(4):203-217. doi: 10.1016/j.aimed.2020.07.004. Epub 2020 Aug 1. PMID: 32837894; PMCID: PMC7395221.

Research:

Aucoin M, Cardozo V, McLaren MD, Garber A, Remy D, Baker J, Gratton A, Kala MA, Monteiro S, Warder C, Perciballi A, Cooley K. A systematic review on the effects of *Echinacea* supplementation on cytokine levels: Is there a role in COVID-19? Metabol Open. 2021 Sep;11:100115. doi:

10.1016/j.metop.2021.100115. Epub 2021 Jul 29. PMID: 34341776; PMCID: PMC8320399.

Licorice Root

Licorice root is an herb that is used in many Chinese herbal formulas. It is used to balance the other herbs in the formula. It is also a natural antiviral. I would not depend on this herb alone to treat a virus. Research indicates it is effective against SARS Covid viruses, but there are many herbs that are more dependable, in my opinion.

Ginger Root

Ginger is not in the category of treating viruses in Western or Chinese medicine, so I would not depend on it. But if it is used in the early stages of a cold, flu, or allergies, it might help. It is a natural anti-inflammatory if taken in a high enough dose. It also increases stomach acid secretion, so it can help with digestive issues. You can either take bulk ginger root capsules, which are available in most stores, or take ginger root extract. The extract enables you to take one pill instead of three or four.

Ginger is a natural anti-inflammatory, and it does reduce blood clotting, although not as strongly as other herbs and enzymes. Please refer to the Blood Clot Prevention chapter.

Ginger root chews and tea are very popular. There is a chance that if you consumed those daily, you would be less likely to contract a viral infection.

Although I would not use ginger root as an antiviral, research indicates it can be used against some viruses. You can also take this daily. It has many functions, and it can be beneficial to take it daily.

The following article discusses how preventing and treating blood clotting issues should be a key part of treating COVID-19.

Research:

Janardhan V, Janardhan V, Kalousek V. COVID-19 as a Blood Clotting Disorder Masquerading as a Respiratory Illness: A Cerebrovascular Perspective and Therapeutic Implications for Stroke Thrombectomy. J Neuroimaging. 2020 Sep;30(5):555-561. doi: 10.1111/jon.12770. Epub 2020 Aug 18. PMID: 32776617; PMCID: PMC7436381.

5

Antiviral Herbal Medicine, Single Chinese Herbs

Chinese herbs are by far the strongest, and most dependable herbs to treat viruses and bacteria. They are often effective at lower doses than other herbs. This chapter is information about single Chinese herbs. There are a few herbs, like Ban Lan Gan, which can be taken by itself as a single herb, but the strongest benefit is when the herb is combined with other antiviral herbs in a formula.

Chinese Antiviral Herbs

Chinese herbs that are used as antivirals are categorized as clearing heat, and relieving toxicity, or clearing toxic heat. The word toxin refers to fevers and other symptoms of infectious diseases, which can be viral or bacterial in origin. These herbs treat inflammation, and infections.

These herbs are listed by their common name first. That is the term most often used in English. Please note that there are often several different herbs that use the same common name, but they are not the same herb.

The Latin or botanical name is important, but even more important for this list is the Chinese name. The Chinese name is very specific to Chinese medicine. Herbs can be processed in different ways which change the energy and function of the herb. In addition, there are different parts of each herb, such as the root, leaf, or flower. Each part of the plant can have a different function.

I have included only the most commonly used, and easy to find herbs. There are thousands of herbs in Chinese medicine, but if you cannot buy them in the West, it won't help you much.

Chinese Herbs are Combined into Formulas

The following Chinese herbs are my first choice to treat viral infections. Information about single herbs, as well as modern research confirming their effectiveness is included. Although Chinese herbs are usually combined in formulas, each herb would work on its own.

This category of herbs is called clearing toxic heat, so the temperature is cool or cold. Chinese medicine theory sees infections as heat. Heat is inflammation, infection, including bacterial and viral infections.

Toxic heat clearing herbs should not be used daily on a long-term basis. They should be used as needed only. The herbs in the prevention chapter can be used more regularly. The reason they should not be used every day forever is that taking an herb that is cold and bitter could affect digestion. I also believe they might impact the good bacteria in the colon. Since these herbs are broad spectrum, you do not have to know which virus or bacteria you are treating.

There is no known instance of viruses becoming immune from the effects of herbs. I also do not know of anyone who suffered from taking these herbs regularly, it is just not the norm. When the COVID-19 pandemic started, I would take antiviral herbs every time I went out in public.

Healthcare Workers

If I worked in a hospital, or was regularly exposed to pathogens, I would probably consider taking these herbs daily for prevention. For prevention, I would probably take one pill several times a day.

For an active infection, taking a full dose every 2-3 hours is important. A digestive upset can be treated with ginger root, which increases stomach acid secretion, and it is a warming herb, which would counterbalance the cold bitter herbs that treat viruses and bacteria.

The herbs listed as using caution while pregnant are oldenlandia, and skullcap. However, I would suggest that pregnant women avoid using herbs of any type, unless prescribed by a qualified herbalist. Instead of herbs, trying high doses of vitamin C would probably be preferable to taking herbs. No one will give advice to pregnant women, because each individual is different, and there is no way to know what underlying issues there are.

Chinese herbs are said to enter meridians, or channels. This often reflects the organ that is impacted, so the herbs that enter the lung channel, also impact the lung organ.

In acupuncture school we learn individual herbs in the second year of school. We pass around the herbs in glass containers and each student takes a sample. We often taste them. If an herb is very strong, you can sometimes feel it in the affected organ. I once tasted an herb that was bitter, that affected the heart meridian, and I felt an immediate sensation in my heart.

Resource for This Chapter

The main source of information for this chapter is the textbook used by acupuncturists in their second year of acupuncture school. *Chinese*

Herbal Medicine Materia Medica. This book was written by Dan Bensky, and Andrew Gamble, with Ted Kaptchuk. This is an excellent book, and if you would like to learn more about Chinese herbs, it is a great reference.

- Most of these herbs are sold under their Chinese names.
- These herbs are not used alone, except for a few herbs.

The Latin names for herbs might vary slightly from what you find online. It might be spelled differently, or be very similar to the Chinese version. For example, licorice root is glycyrrhiza glabra in America, and glycyrrhiza uralensis in China. That is why the Chinese name should be deferred to for accuracy.

The following table is a quick reference to Chinese herbs in the clear toxic heat category. They are explained more fully below.

Research Notes

Normally research references are placed in the back of the book. I have chosen to include the references I used immediately after each herb or herbal formula.

Modern research on single herbs is easier to find than research on formulas. These herbs are combined with other herbs to make a formula. There are infinite names for formulas. A formula could be made tomorrow with a brand-new name, and it could be marketed as a proprietary formula in China.

These herbs are sold over the counter and online. Each herb company will make slight alterations to the formula, based on what their herbalist prefers.

Andrographis

Andrographis, Chuan Xin Lian, Herba Andrographitis paniculatae
Properties: Bitter, cold
Channels entered: Large intestine, Lung, Small Intestine, Stomach
Functions: Clears heat and fire toxicity. Clears lung inflammation, and sore throat caused by infection. It is also used in a formula called Chuan Xin Lian to treat bladder infections, and most types of infection can benefit from this formula.
Products: Nature's Way, Planetary Herbals, and Solaray make Andrographis extracts.

Andrographis is a Top Herb for Viruses and Bacteria

Andrographis is perhaps the most studied antiviral herb. This would be my first choice for a single herb to fight bacteria or viruses, although I would prefer to take the Chinese herbal formula called Chuan Xin Lian. This is a formula would be very helpful to keep around to use as needed. I have used it to treat many different types of infections, both viral and bacterial.

The brand I use is available only through licensed acupuncturists, Golden Flower Chinese Herbs. Their formula is called Andrographis. It contains andrographis, isatis root, and dandelion. Other companies also make this formula.

Andrographis and Ban Lan Gen (Isatis Root) are my top choices to take in a pinch, if you cannot get a complete herbal formula. Many companies have an andrographis product.

Paradise Herbs has a product that has, per two capsules: 400 mg. andrographis extract, plus isatis root, lonicera (honeysuckle), and elderberry. I have not used this product, but it has a good combination of antivirals.

Nature's Way has an andrographis with 300 mg. andrographis extract, plus 100 mg. of other parts of the plant, per capsule. Planetary Herbals makes a Full Spectrum Andrographis Extract, with 300 mg. andrographis extract, plus 100 mg. of other andrographis parts, per tablet.

Research:

> Mandal A, Jha AK, Hazra B. Plant Products as Inhibitors of Coronavirus 3CL Protease. Front Pharmacol. 2021 Mar 9;12:583387. doi: 10.3389/fphar.2021.583387. PMID: 33767619; PMCID: PMC7985176.

Research:

> Enmozhi SK, Raja K, Sebastine I, Joseph J. Andrographolide as a potential inhibitor of SARS-CoV-2 main protease: an in silico approach. *J Biomol Struct Dyn*. 2021;39(9):3092-3098. doi:10.1080/07391102.2020.1760136

Forsythia Fruit

Forsythia fruit, Lian Qiao, Fructus forsythia suspensae

Properties: Bitter, slightly acrid, cool

Channels entered: Heart, Liver, Gallbladder

Functions: Clears toxic heat. Can be used for neck lumps, nodules, and boils caused by infection.

Research:

> Xiong, X., Wang, P., Su, K., Cho, W. C., & Xing, Y. (2020). Chinese herbal medicine for coronavirus disease 2019: A systematic review and meta-

analysis. *Pharmacological research*, *160*, 105056. https://doi.org/10.1016/j.phrs.2020.105056

Honeysuckle Flower

Honeysuckle flower, Jin Yin Hua, Lonicera
Properties: Sweet, cold
Channels entered: Large intestine, Lung, Stomach
Date recorded: Tang Materia Medica in 659 AD
Functions: Clears heat and fire toxicity. Clears damp heat from the lower burner (large intestines).

Research:

Alice Grigore, Daniel Cord, Cristiana Tanase & Radu Albulescu (2020) Herbal medicine, a reliable support in COVID therapy, Journal of Immunoassay and Immunochemistry, 41:6, 976-999, DOI: 10.1080/15321819.2020.1862867

Another research article stated that "Lonicera was verified to inhibit influenza viral replication in vitro and in vivo."

Research:

Xiong Y, Li NX, Duan N, Liu B, Zhu H, Zhang C, Li L, Lu C, Huang L. Traditional Chinese Medicine in Treating Influenza: From Basic Science to Clinical Applications. Front Pharmacol. 2020 Sep 15;11:575803. doi: 10.3389/fphar.2020.575803. PMID: 33041821; PMCID: PMC7526665.

The article referenced above also states that "In addition to the direct effect on the influenza virus, TCM regulates immune activation and signaling pathways that impact on the influenza virus." TCM is an abbreviation of Traditional Chinese Medicine.

It also states that "Several experiments have confirmed that TCM is the most potent anti-inflammatory natural medicine which can modulate all kinds of cytokines and immune molecules."

They tested Coptis, Isatis, Lonicera, Scutellaria baicalensis, Cyrtomium fortunei, Houttuynia cordata, Gardenia jasminoides, and Chrysanthemum.

Cyrtomium fortunei is the only herb not mentioned elsewhere in this book. The information I found was that it was a type of Holly. This underlines how important it is to include the Chinese name for the herb. There are probably many types of Holly. This is listed as Ping Wu online. It is not included in my herb references.

Dandelion

Dandelion, Pu Gong Ying, Herba taraxaci,
Properties: Bitter, sweet, cold
Channels entered: Liver, Stomach

Historical Use Record: Tang Materia Medica in 659 AD

Functions: Clears heat, and fire toxicity. It reduces abscesses, and nodules. It also promotes lactation when the lactation problem is caused by inflammation, or infection.

Notes: This herb is commonly used to cleanse the liver in Western herbalism. It is combined with several other herbs in a formula called Chuan Xin Lian, which is used to treat bladder infections.

Since dandelion can be taken daily long term, and it cleanses the blood, and regulates the liver and gallbladder, this is a good option to take daily for an extended period of time.

While I would not depend on dandelion as a single herb to treat an acute infection, it does have many benefits and no known downside of regular consumption.

Dandelion benefits the liver and gallbladder, which improves digestion, and treats fatigue caused by liver imbalances. I would take 1,000 mg. three times per day. I have not been able to find a dandelion extract as a single herb. It is best to combine dandelion with other herbs.

There are many liver cleansing herbal formulas available. Planetary Herbals Bupleurum Liver Cleanse is a great formula. It combines Western and Chinese herbs to regulate and heal the liver. If you would like to take dandelion extract as a single herb, you can either drink a cleansing tea, dandelion tea, or buy the herbal extract under the name Pu Gong Ying.

Research:

Common dandelion (*Taraxacum officinale*) efficiently blocks the interaction between ACE2 cell surface receptor and SARS-CoV-2 spike protein D614, mutants D614G, N501Y, K417N and E484K *in vitro* Hoai Thi Thu Tran, Nguyen Phan Khoi Le, Michael Gigl, Corinna Dawid, Evelyn Lamy bioRxiv 2021.03.19.435959; doi: https://doi.org/10.1101/2021.03.19.435959

Forsythia

Forsythia fruit, Fructus forsythia suspensae, Lian Qiao
Properties: Bitter, slightly acrid, and cool
Channels: Heart, Liver, and Gallbladder
This herb is not taken alone. It is used in multiple herbal formulas.

Research:

Ren, Wei et al. "Research progress of traditional Chinese medicine against COVID-19." *Biomedicine & pharmacotherapy = Biomedecine & pharmacotherapie* vol. 137 (2021): 111310. doi:10.1016/j.biopha.2021.111310

Houttuynia

Houttuynia, Yu Xing Cao, Herba cum radice houttuyniae cordatae
Functions: Clears heat and toxin, and dissipates nodules.
Properties: Acrid, cool
Channels: Large Intestine, Lung
Functions: Clears toxic heat, and treats lung abscesses, lung heat cough, with thick yellow sputum. Used internally and externally for toxic sores.

Although this herb is primarily used in formulas, not taken alone, due to the popularity of Chinese antiviral herbs, I have noticed some companies are making this available as an herbal extract single herb. It is listed under its Chinese name as Yu Xing Cao.

Research:

Bahadur Gurung A, Ajmal Ali M, Lee J, Abul Farah M, Mashay Al-Anazi K, Al-Hemaid F. Identification of SARS-CoV-2 inhibitors from extracts of *Houttuynia cordata* Thunb. Saudi J Biol Sci. 2021 Sep 6. doi: 10.1016/j.sjbs.2021.08.100. Epub ahead of print. PMID: 34512097; PMCID: PMC8420092.

Isatis Leaf

Isatis, Woad leaf, indigo, Da Qing Ye, Folium Daqingye
Properties: bitter, very cold
Channels: Heart, Lung, Stomach
Functions: Clears toxic heat. Treats any disease which causes fever, severe contagious diseases. Treats throat and lung fire toxin (inflammation). Treats red skin blotches due to internal heat.

Research:

> Mandal A, Jha AK, Hazra B. Plant Products as Inhibitors of Coronavirus 3CL Protease. Front Pharmacol. 2021 Mar 9;12:583387. doi: 10.3389/fphar.2021.583387. PMID: 33767619; PMCID: PMC7985176.

Isatis Root

Isatis, Woad root, Ban Lan Gen, Radix Isatidid sue Baphicacanthi
Properties: bitter, cold
Channels: Heart, Lung, Stomach
Functions: treats toxic heat, cools the blood, treats sore throat from infections. Can be used for mumps and jaundice.

Notes: Notice this is the root portion of the isatis plant. This herb is often available over the counter as a product combined with sugar and made into a tea.

Ban Lan Gen Keli is a popular herbal product. This product is isatis root powder combined with sugar and packaged in little sachets to be mixed with hot water. If you would like to buy an herbal extract powder, try the Chinese name of Ban Lan Gen. Since this herb is commonly used as a single herb in China, there are a lot of products available.

Ban Lan Gen products are often made with sugar, which offsets the bitter taste of the herb. You can barely taste the herb when it is combined with sugar in these prepared packets. It is not hard to get someone to take this herb in that form. Simply put the herbal powder into a mug, and combine with hot water.

Research:

> Yu, Bin et al. "Network pharmacology study on the mechanism of the Chinese medicine Radix Isatidis (Banlangen) for COVID-19." *Medicine* vol. 100,32 (2021): e26881. doi:10.1097/MD.0000000000026881

This article elaborates on how Ban Lan Gen, or isatis root, has been used to treat mumps, erysipelas, carbuncle sores, bacteria, cancer, viral hepatitis, respiratory viral infections, and viral skin diseases.

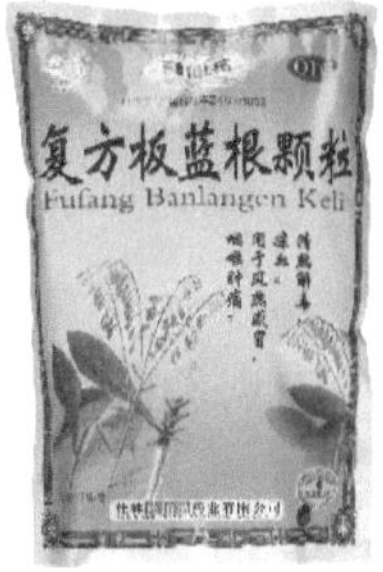

Southern Ban Lan Gen

There will always be brands and products available online, which cannot all be listed in a book, because these herbs are big business in China, and there are dozens of herb companies making herbs to sell over the counter. You just need to look at the ingredients. You will recognize the antiviral herbs listed in this chapter. These products might also have herbs not listed in this book, because they might not be commonly used in America.

I came across this product, called Southern Ban Lan Gen. It contains Ban Lan Gen, which is Isatis root, with Pu Gong Ying, which is dandelion root, with Viola, which is another antiviral herb.

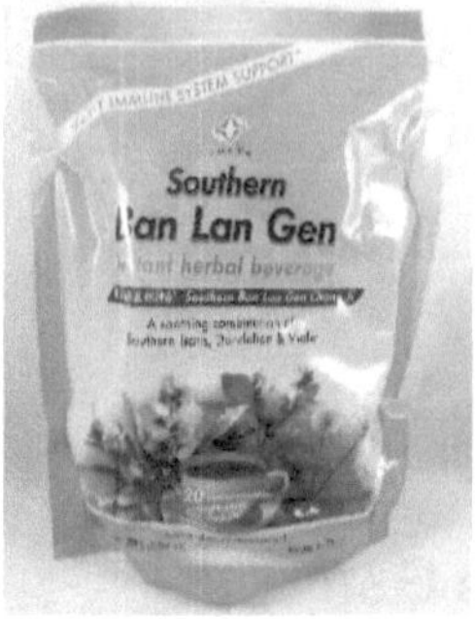

This is how Ban Lan Gen tea looks:

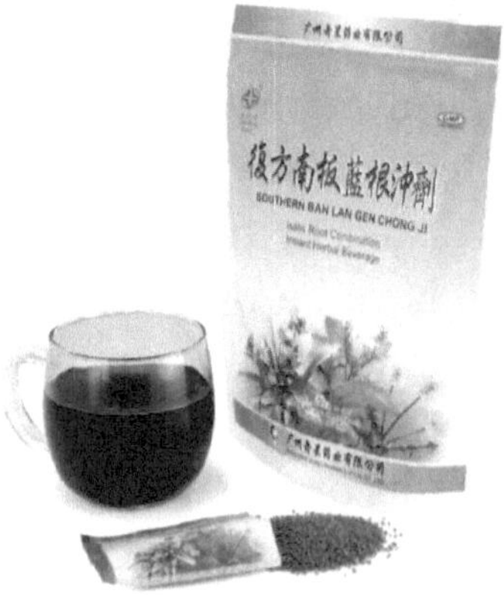

Oldenlandia

Oldenlandia, Bai Hua She She Cao, Herba hedyotidis diffusae

Properties: Bitter, sweet, cold

Channels: Liver, Stomach, Large Intestine

Functions: Clears toxic heat, reduces abscesses. Promotes urination to clear heat. Used for intestinal abscesses.

Research:

Zheng, Y., Jin, D., Lin, J., Zhang, Y., Tian, J., Lian, F., & Tong, X. (2021). Understanding COVID-19 in Wuhan From the Perspective of Cold-Dampness: Clinical Evidences and Mechanisms. *Frontiers in medicine*, *8*, 617659. https://doi.org/10.3389/fmed.2021.617659

Viola

Viola, Yedeon's violet, Zi Hua Di Ding, Herba cum radice violae yedoensitis

Properties: Acrid, bitter, cold

Channels: Heart, Liver

Functions: Clears toxic heat. Good for red eyes sore throat, and mumps.

Research for Viola was primarily for treating bacterial infections. Most herbs that treat bacterial infections also treat viruses.

Research:

Wong, R. W., Hägg, U., Samaranayake, L., Yuen, M. K., Seneviratne, C. J., & Kao, R. (2010). Antimicrobial activity of Chinese medicine herbs against common bacteria in oral biofilm. A pilot study. *International journal of oral and maxillofacial surgery*, *39*(6), 599–605. https://doi.org/10.1016/j.ijom.2010.02.024

Wild Chrysanthemum Flower

Wild Chrysanthemum flower, Ye Ju Hua, Flos chrysanthemi indici
Properties: bitter, acrid, slightly cold
Channels: Lung, Liver
Functions: Clears toxic heat, sore threat, sores on body.

Research:

Mahmoudi S, Balmeh N, Mohammadi N, Sadeghian-Rizi T. The Novel Drug Discovery to Combat COVID-19 by Repressing Important Virus Proteins Involved in Pathogenesis Using Medicinal Herbal Compounds. Avicenna J Med Biotechnol. 2021 Jul-Sep;13(3):107-115. doi: 10.18502/ajmb.v13i3.6370. PMID: 34484639; PMCID: PMC8377408.

Skullcap Root, Scutellaria, Scute

Skullcap root, Scutellaria, Scute, Huang Qin, Radix scutellaria baicalensis.
This herb is called Chinese skullcap by some authors.
Properties: bitter, cold
Channels: Gallbladder, Large intestine, Lung, Stomach

Functions: Clears fire and heat in the lung. Stops bleeding, treats nosebleed.
Notes: This herb is in the damp heat clearing category, not the toxic heat category. It is usually combined with other herbs to treat viruses.

Although some authors reference this as Chinese skullcap and highly recommend it for viruses, I have not tried it alone. Recently there are more products available. If you wanted to take it as a single herb, you could also find it under the Chinese name Huang Qin.

Research:

Liu H, Ye F, Sun Q, Liang H, Li C, Li S, Lu R, Huang B, Tan W, Lai L. *Scutellaria baicalensis* extract and baicalein inhibit replication of SARS-CoV-2 and its 3C-like protease *in vitro*. J Enzyme Inhib Med Chem. 2021 Dec;36(1):497-503. doi: 10.1080/14756366.2021.1873977. PMID: 33491508; PMCID: PMC7850424.

Wormwood

Wormwood, Qing Hao, Herba Artemisiae Annuae.
Properties: bitter, cold
Channels: Kidney, Liver, Gallbladder
Functions: Clears heat, treats malaria, and chills and fever of malaria.

Wormwood is very effective to kill parasites. It is used as an antiviral herb in Chinese medicine.

It is always combined with other antiviral herbs in formulas.

Research:

Fuzimoto AD. An overview of the anti-SARS-CoV-2 properties of Artemisia annua, its antiviral action, protein-associated mechanisms, and repurposing for COVID-19 treatment. J Integr Med. 2021 Sep;19(5):375-388. doi: 10.1016/j.joim.2021.07.003. Epub 2021 Jul 22. PMID: 34479848; PMCID: PMC8378675.

Wormwood is a Chinese herb that was traditionally used for thousands of years to treat malarial disorders. It has been used by many countries to treat parasites. Malaria is caused by a parasite, so if natural substances were to be used, wormwood would be a good choice.

For an active infection, I would not recommend wormwood as a single herb. I do not know if it is not strong enough by itself to protect you. It is always combined with other herbs in Chinese medicine herbal formulas to treat viruses.

I wanted to draw the correlation between how wormwood is used all over the world to treat parasites, and how it can also be used to treat some viruses. It is an herb in the Chinese formula Zhong Gan Ling, which is one of my favorite antiviral formulas. This is explained in the chapter on Chinese herbal formulas.

There is a lot of interest in the scientific community on whether this herb can be used to treat viruses. Of course, it has already been used to treat viruses in Chinese medicine.

Research:

"A. annua constituents may impede the SARS-CoV-2 attachment, membrane fusion, internalization into the host cells, and hinder the viral replication and transcription process. "

This quote is from a recent study. It implies that the SARS and Covid viruses are not able to attach to the cells as well when wormwood has been administered. This also slows down the virus growth in the body.

There are hundreds of antiviral herbs. This is just one of them, as you have seen from this book. Treating viruses is routine in Chinese medicine. It is very frustrating knowing that there are so many antiviral herbs, but most people are suffer needlessly.

Research:

Fuzimoto AD. An overview of the anti-SARS-CoV-2 properties of Artemisia annua, its antiviral action, protein-associated mechanisms, and repurposing for COVID-19 treatment. J Integr Med. 2021 Sep;19(5):375-388. doi: 10.1016/j.joim.2021.07.003. Epub 2021 Jul 22. PMID: 34479848; PMCID: PMC8378675.

6

Chinese Herbal Formulas, the Most Powerful Choice

The herbal formulas in this chapter are the strongest herbal antiviral formulas. In my opinion, there is no stronger herbal supplement on the market.

There are dozens of herbal formulas to treat viral and bacterial infections. They contain herbs that are in the "clear toxic heat" category. Other herbs can be combined with these formulas to boost the immune system.

Companies that manufacture Chinese herbal medicine often have slightly different formulations. They might add an herb or two, or change the amounts of each herb in the formula.

For an active infection, whether it is viral or bacterial, or unknown, it is usually more effective to take about 1,000 mg. every two hours. Since viral infections can kill you, it is usually advised to treat early and often. If in doubt, treat, and treat several days past the time you think the virus is active.

Chinese Herb Shortages During Flu Season

Every flu season there are shortages of Chinese herbal medicine to treat viruses. It is a good idea to buy your herbs in advance. If you find yourself with a shortage of herbs, take one pill every two hours. Each pill should be about 500 mg.

If you can only find Chinese Teapills, which are patented pellet herbs, they are not as strong, so you will need to take 6-8 pills. These pellets are mixed with honey.

I would not depend on the pellets to get rid of COVID-19. If you can only get pellets, you would be better off buying a single herbal extract like Ban Lan Gen, and taking that every two hours.

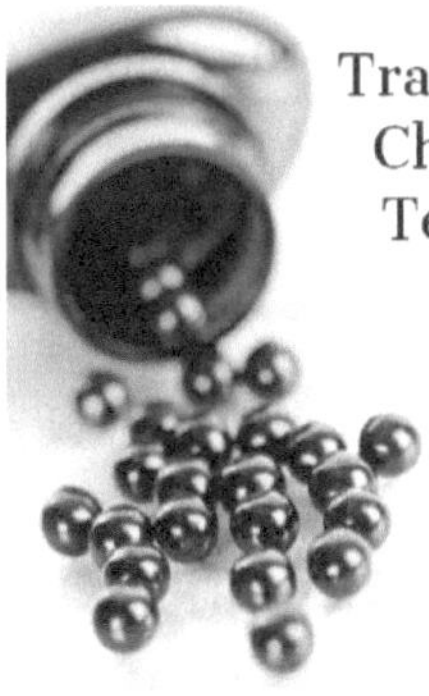

Traditional Chinese Teapills

Spread out your dosage, taking smaller amounts more often. This is the best use of the herbs. Chinese herbs are the most effective antivirals available. The average flu will be fully treated within two days in most cases. The sooner you catch it, the easier it is to get rid of.

I would combine Chinese herbs with hourly doses of 1 gram of vitamin C. That is the best thing you can do to treat a virus. This will keep your blood levels of vitamin C and antiviral herbs stable throughout the day, making them both more effective. If you take your vitamin C hourly, it is easy to take 1,000 mg. That is just two tablets.

If you do not get rapid results within 24 hours of starting Chinese herbs for the flu, I would consider adding an immune tonic, like cordyceps, Jade Windscreen, or astragalus extract. These are explained in the Prevention chapter. Antiviral herbs stop the virus from taking over, but your immune system still has to be strong enough to fight it off, as well as recover from the damage that is done.

Most Powerful Antiviral:

Chinese Herbal Medicine
+ Vitamin C, 1 gram per hour
+ Cordyceps

Your first choice is to find a local acupuncturist, who is certified in Chinese herbs, and get their help.

I did a survey of what products were easy to buy online. Golden Flower Chinese Herbs is only available through acupuncturists, so to give you a good idea of dependable brands, I will list my choice in order:

1. Golden Flower Chinese Herbs
2. Kan Traditionals
3. Guang Ci Tang
4. Dr. Shen's

I have not personally used the Dr. Shen's brand of herbs. I have acupuncturist friends who use the Guang Ci Tang brand. This brand appears to not be made into teapills, so it is not mixed with honey.

I do not personally like the Plum Flower brand pellets, due to past experience. Some brands are not very strong.

You should feel a difference within 24 hours, if not a few hours. That is a good test of the quality. You can also test by smell. If the herbs do not smell strong when you open the bottle, they might not be good quality.

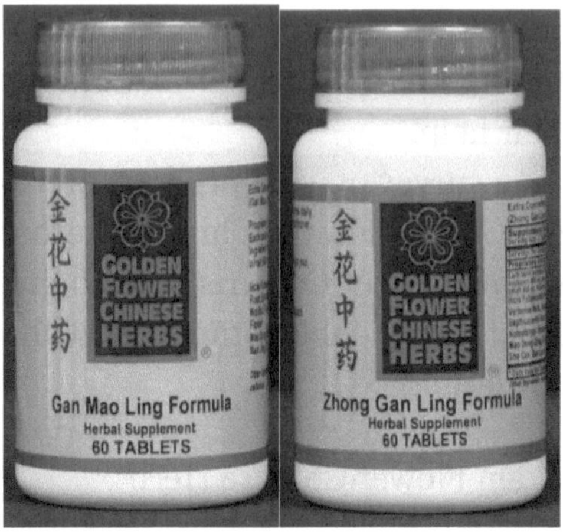
金花中药
GOLDEN FLOWER CHINESE HERBS
Gan Mao Ling Formula
Herbal Supplement
60 TABLETS
金花中药
GOLDEN FLOWER CHINESE HERBS
Zhong Gan Ling Formula
Herbal Supplement
60 TABLETS

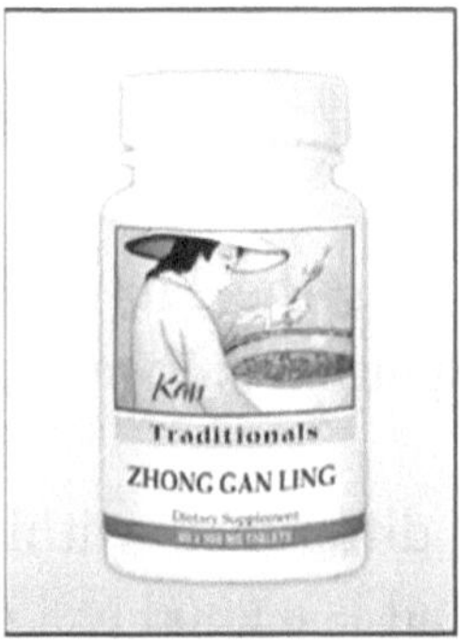
Traditionals
ZHONG GAN LING

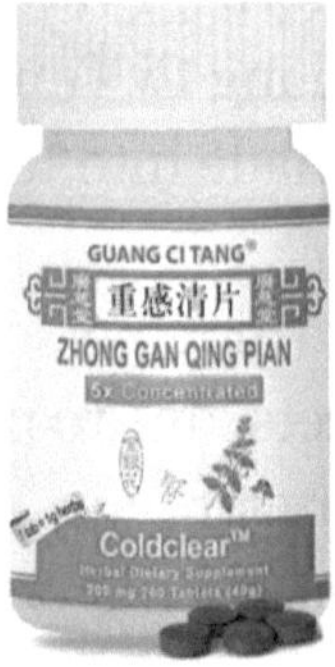
GUANG CI TANG®
重感清片
ZHONG GAN QING PIAN
5x Concentrated
Coldclear™

Antiviral herbs can be
taken every two hours
as needed for infections

Zhong Gan Ling

My personal favorite formula to treat viruses is Zhong Gan Ling. Every acupuncturist will have preferred formulas to treat viruses. They might use a completely different formula. Both Gan Mao Ling, and Zhong Gan Ling are very popular to treat all types of viruses.

These formulas usually sell out at the onset of every cold and flu season, so stocking up in advance is advised. The herbs will be effective for a long time. Although I try to keep my herbs fresh, I would not hesitate to use Chinese herbs that have been stored for many years.

Zhong Gan Ling is a patent formula. This means that many companies make a version of this formula. The Chinese government wanted to know which herbs were strongest for use against viruses, and they developed these two modern formulas, Gan Mao Ling, and Zhong Gan Ling.

Golden Flower Chinese Herbs carries the following formula:

- Holly root, Ilex, Mao Dong Qing, Ilicis Pubescentis Radix – 19%
- Kudzu root, Ge Gen, Pueraria Radix – 19.6%
- Isatis leaf, Indigo Woad Leaf, Da Qing Ye, Isatidis folium
- Verbena, Ma Bian Cao, Verbenae Herba – 13%
- Oldenlandia, Bai Hua She She Cao, Hedyotis Diffusae Herba – 13%
- Isatis root, Ban Lan Gen, Isatidis seu Baphicacanthis radix – 10%
- Sweet wormwood, Qing Hao, Artemisiae Annuae Herba – 5%
- Gypsum, Shi Gao, Gypsum Fibrosum – 3%
- Notopterygium, Qiang Huo, Notopterygii rhizome seu Radix – 2%

Zhong Gan Ling

Mao Dong Qing 19.6%	Ban Lan Gen 10.1%
Ge Gen 19.6%	Qing Hao 5%
Da Qing Ye 14.6%	Shi Gao 2.9%
Ma Bian Cao 13%	Qiang Huo 2.2%
Bai Hua She She Cao 13%	

Golden Flower Chinese Herbs

Zhong Gan Ling herbs listed with the common herb names.

Zhong Gan Ling	English names
Holly root 19.6%	Isatis root 10.1%
Kudzu root 19.6%	Sweet wormwood 5%
Isatis leaf 14.6%	Gypsum 2.9%
Verbena 13%	Notopterygium 2.2%
Oldenlandia 13%	

Golden Flower Chinese Herbs

Every company that makes this might have a slightly different ingredient list. The most important thing to look for is that their formula is very similar to these.

Zhong Gan Ling can be used for:

- Bronchitis
- Common cold
- Fever
- Flu
- Swollen lymph nodes
- Cough
- Sore throat
- Strep throat

I always try to get my patients to keep a bottle of this formula handy, in case they need it. I have used it on my dad, who is in his eighties. He was coming down with the flu and this formula got rid of it in two doses. I caught it on the first day, which is always the key. If he had waited a few days, it would have taken him two to three days of herbs to get over the virus.

If he had not responded quickly to the antiviral formula, I might have also added cordyceps to boost his immune system and help him get rid of the virus faster. This flu infection happened prior to the current pandemic infection. I would not stop taking antiviral herbs until I had been symptom free for five days or longer. The common cold or flu has easier symptoms to recognize, and it is easier to get rid of.

Now, I would also combine these herbs with high doses of vitamin C. The more things you can throw at a virus, the better, in my opinion. It is war, and you have to act fast.

Chuan Xin Lian

This formula is also called andrographis formula. It is a strong antiviral and antibacterial formula. This is one of the best formulas to take, if someone wanted to take something long term, such as overcoming latent infections, or serious illness. As mentioned before, this is a popular formula to treat bladder infections, and I use it to treat most types of infections.

Dozens of companies make this formula, and it is easy to find online.

Andrographis, Chuan Xin Lian – 50%
Isatis root, Ban Lan Gen – 25%
Dandelion, Pu Gong Ying – 25%

Chuan Xin Lian
Andrographis Formula

Andrographis, Chuan Xin Lian – 50%
Isatis root, Ban Lan Gen – 25%
Dandelion, Pu Gong Ying – 25%

Golden Flower Chinese Herbs

As you can see from this long list, Chuan Xin Lian formula can be very helpful to have around, to use as needed. It treats bacteria, viruses, and is anti-fever, and anti-inflammatory. To confirm, with modern research, the benefits of these herbs, you would need to research each herb individually. If you understand that these diseases are caused by viruses and bacteria, which Chinese medicine views as toxic heat, it makes sense. Herb companies, even ones that make Chinese herbs, are not allowed to make medical claims of curing diseases, and I am not doing that here.

Chuan Xin Lian
can be used for:

Bladder infections
Bronchitis
Chicken pox
Common cold
Dysentery
Ear infections
Fever
Flu
Gastroenteritis
Gum infection
Hepatitis
Herpes simplex and zoster
Kidney infection
Laryngitis
Lung infections
Measles
Mumps
Pelvic inflammatory disease
Sinus infection or inflammation
Skin infections
Sore throat
Strep throat
Tonsillitis

Gan Mao Ling

Gan Mao Ling is an example of a more modern formula to treat colds and flu, and other viruses that attack the lungs. The ingredients are:

- Holly root, Ilex, Mao Dong Qing, Ilicis Pubescentis Radix – 25%
- Isatis root, Ban Lan Gen, Isatidis seu Baphicacanthis radix – 20%
- Evodia root, San Ya Ku, Evodiae Radix – 20%

- Chrysanthemum, Ju Hua, Chrysanthemi flos – 13%
- Vitex fruit, Man Jing Zi, Viticis Fructus - 12%
- Honeysuckle flower, Jin Yin Hua, Lonicerae flos – 10%

The top two herbs are holly and isatis. Isatis is called Ban Lan Gen in Chinese. This herb is sold over the counter in a single herb product. You can buy the herb in an extract of 100-gram container, which is the pure herb. Ban Lan Gen Keli, or similar products are combined with sugar. When this bitter herb is combined with sugar, it does not taste bitter at all.

Gan Mao Ling clears toxic heat, soothes the throat to stop coughing, and opens the sinuses. According to Dr. Jake Fratkin, it is the number one selling herbal formula in China. It is sold over the counter and commonly used to treat diseases caused by viral infections.

Gan Mao Ling

Holly root, Ilex, Mao Dong Qing – 25%
Isatis root, Ban Lan Gen – 20%
Evodia root, San Ya Ku – 20%
Chrysanthemum, Ju Hua – 13%
Vitex fruit, Man Jing Zi - 12%
Honeysuckle flower, Jin Yin Hua – 10%

Golden Flower Chinese Herbs

Gan Mao Ling can be used for:

- Cold
- Ear infection
- Fever
- Flu
- Headache
- Measles, early stage
- Sinus congestion
- Sinus infection
- Sore throat
- Tonsillitis

I have compared Golden Flower Chinese Herbs, which is available only through acupuncturists, with the Dr. Shen formula. It appears the formulas are very similar.

This is how I compare herbal formulas as an herbalist. I look at each herb in the formula, and see what percentage each herb is in the formula. If I need a replacement for Golden Flower Gan Mao Ling, I would choose something similar.

Gan Mao Ling, Golden Flower, Percentage of formula		**Gan Mao Ling, Dr. Shen, by Mg.**	
Pin Yin	Pct	Pin Yin	Amount
Mao Dong Qing	35.00%	Mao Dong Qing	703 mg.
Ban Lan Gen	16.00%	Ban Lan Gen	273 mg.
Wu Zhu Yu	13.00%	Wu Zhu Yu	462 mg
Ju Hua	13.00%	Ju Hua	273 mg.
Man Jing Zi	13.00%	Man Jing Zi	273 mg.
Jin Yin Hua	10.00%	Jin Yin Hua	105 mg.

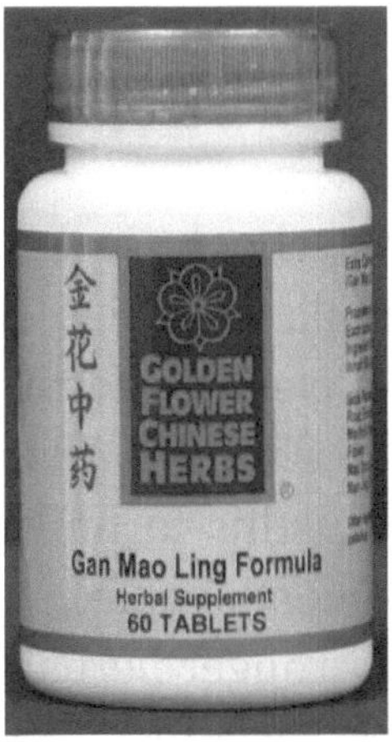

Purchasing Chinese Herbs

Activeherb.com carries numerous brands of Chinese herbs, and I like how their website explains each herb in the formula and how it is traditionally used. Dr. Shen formulas can be found at www.drshen.com. The herbs are explained as clearing heat and toxins in Chinese medicine.

Herb companies must be careful to not say they treat disease with herbs, everything must be explained in Chinese medicine terms. I have included the research that has been done on the individual herbs, verifying that the single herbs are antiviral, so that solves that problem.

Yin Qiao San

In acupuncture school we learned about using the herbal formula Yin Qiao San to treat colds and flu. This is a classical formula and it is sold over the counter in China. I will not include a lot of information about this formula, because it does not work well for most people.

We have much stronger herbal formulas to treat viruses these days. I wanted to mention it, as you will probably see this formula listed, or a variation of it online if you do research on Chinese herbal medicine. Yin Qiao Jie Du Pian is a variation of this formula, and I'm sure it does work for some people, but I have never had success with it, and I personally use other formulas.

Favorite Brands of Chinese Herbs

My first choice of brands for Chinese herbal medicine is Golden Flower Chinese Herbs. This brand is only available through licensed acupuncturists. Golden Flower makes pharmaceutical grade herbs in tablet form. I have been using this brand since 1996, and I always find them to be the most effective.

Golden Flower also carries jumbo bottles of 240 tablets. This is a good option to keep around to treat a family. I have kept Golden Flower herb bottles which are over 10 years old. They are still very effective.

Herbs don't expire like drugs, or even vitamins, which can degrade over time. It is worth the extra money and effort to use the strongest herbs you can buy.

Chinese herbal extracts are available in powder form, and KPC is my first choice. This brand is usually only available through acupuncturists also. Although I would recommend you find an acupuncturist who will help you stock up on Zhong Gan Ling, or Gan Mao Ling made by Golden Flower. This might not be an option for you.

Modern Chinese Antiviral Resource

In acupuncture school we learn what are called classical formulas. These herbal formulas have been used for thousands of years. However, Chinese medicine is always evolving.

A great resource for information on antiviral herbs is Dr. Jake Fratkin. He has written numerous articles on Chinese herbs and modern usage. His website is www.DrJakeFratkin.com.

Dr. Fratkin said that Gan Mao Ling is the number one selling herbal formula in China. I have used his website as a much-appreciated resource in my study of antiviral herbs, and all things Chinese medicine. He has almost 100 free health articles on his website.

Modern Research on Chinese Herbal Formulas

In response to the COVID-19 virus, new herbal formulas have been developed, that address the symptoms of this virus. There are dozens of formulas, and from what I understand, each hospital was trying different formulas to treat all aspects of this disease. Each phase of the disease could require a different herbal combination. This is used in hospitals, and each patient will have a formula specifically for him or her.

Jin Hua Qing Gan

This formula was studied in China from January 24 to February 17, 2020 on 80 patients. Of the 80 patients, 44 took the herbal formula. This formula is listed in the research as Jinhua Qinggan. The people who took this formula experienced a faster resolution of the virus, as shown by testing. The treated group recovery time was seven to twelve days. The patients who did not receive the herbal formula took ten to 14 days to recover.

Pneumonia

In this study pneumonia recovery time was also reduced in people who took Jin Hua Qing Gan. The patients who took the herbs recovered from pneumonia faster at 8-12 days. The control group, with no herbal treatment, took 10-15 days.

Research:

Liu Z, Li X, Gou C, Li L, Luo X, Zhang C, Zhang Y, Zhang J, Jin A, Li H, Zeng Y, Li T, Wang X. Effect of Jinhua Qinggan granules on novel coronavirus pneumonia in patients. J Tradit Chin Med. 2020 Jun;40(3):467-472. doi: 10.19852/j.cnki.jtcm.2020.03.016. PMID: 32506862.

Dosage

It appears the dosage was given just twice a day, morning and evening, for seven days. In treating serious viruses, I believe a more aggressive plan would have worked faster. I would have suggested taking antiviral herbs every two to three hours, at a minimum.

The herbs in this formula are similar to the ones used in the formulas I already mentioned. The medical experts referred to more than 100 ancient prescriptions in TCM classics such as the Treatise on Febrile Diseases.

They combined the formulas Ma Xing Shi Gan and Yin Qiao San, giving them the following formula:

- Jin Yin Hua, Honeysuckle
- Ma Huang, (this is not sold in America, due to the ephedra content)
- Shi Gao, Gypsum
- Ku Xing Ren, Apricot seed
- Huang Qin, Scutellaria
- Lian Qiao, Forsythia
- Zhe Bei Mu, Fritillaria
- Zhi Mu, Anemarrhena
- Niu Bang Zi, Burdock seed
- Qing Hao, Wormwood
- Bo He, Mint
- Gan Cao, licorice root

7

Vitamin C Made Effective

This might be the most important chapter in this book. Although I have been using herbs for over 20 years to treat viruses, I have only fairly recently discovered how effective high doses of vitamin C can be.

Most people are familiar with using extra vitamin C during a cold or flu to boost the immune system, and resolve the infection faster. They are not getting the results they seek, because they are not taking enough. When you have an active infection, your body quickly uses up its stores of vitamin C. Your body uses vitamin C to fight infections.

Vitamin C is safe and effective, and can be taken daily to boost the immune system, and clear viruses and bacteria.

How Does Vitamin C Work?

An easy way to explain how vitamin C treats disease is that it neutralizes viral and bacterial toxins. It is an antioxidant.

Research:

Kim Y, Kim H, Bae S, Choi J, Lim SY, Lee N, Kong JM, Hwang YI, Kang JS, Lee WJ. Vitamin C Is an Essential Factor on the Anti-viral Immune Responses through the Production of Interferon-α/β at the Initial Stage of Influenza A Virus (H3N2) Infection. Immune Netw. 2013 Apr;13(2):70-4. doi: 10.4110/in.2013.13.2.70. Epub 2013 Apr 30. PMID: 23700397; PMCID: PMC3659258.

There are 263 research articles on PubMed about COVID-19 and vitamin C. A search for "viruses and vitamin C" gives you 873 results. "Antiviral and vitamin C" gives you 1,040 results. There is already ample research about vitamin C and viruses.

In doing research on chronic fatigue, I came across the book, *The Infection Game*, by Dr. Sarah Myhill, and Craig Robinson. Dr. Myhill is a medical doctor in the UK who specializes in treating chronic fatigue. She has her patients change their diet, and take supplements, including high doses of vitamin C, and they recover from chronic fatigue.

This book was groundbreaking for me in understanding how prevalent viral, and bacterial infections are in chronic disease. I have come to the conclusion that many common diseases that are considered to be incurable, are in fact caused by viruses and bacteria, which are fairly easy to treat with natural medicine.

> The patient should get large doses of vitamin C in all pathological conditions while the physician ponders the diagnosis.
>
> Dr. Frederick Robert Klenner, BS MS MD FCCP FAAFP (1907 – 1984)

I will quote Dr. Myhill, from her book, *The Infection Game*:

- "Vitamin C is the most powerful, broad-spectrum antimicrobial that we have available to us. It is completely safe to human cells, with no known toxicity.
- We should be taking at least 5,000 mg., that is 5 grams, of vitamin C daily.
- Vitamin C and sugar also compete for absorption in bacteria, yeasts and cancer cells. Starve these cells of sugar, feed them with vitamin C instead, and you kill them.
- Vitamin C kills viruses on contact.

Taking super-high doses of vitamin C during an infection:

- Directly kills all microbes on contact
- Mitigates any friendly-fire damage by the immune system
- Mops up the free radicals inevitably produced as energy delivery mechanisms are increased."

Notice how she says that it mitigates any friendly fire damage by the immune system?

Perhaps this would help with the intense cytokine storm that is believed to be an important cause of death with COVID-19 patients.

I will not continue quoting her, you should just buy this excellent book.

> Vitamin C
> Kills Viruses
> on Contact

Do Not Heat Vitamin C Above 160 F Degrees

Vitamin C should not be put in boiling water. If the water is over 160 F degrees, the vitamin C will be damaged, and it will not work.

Making Vitamin C Work

In order for Vitamin C to work against pathogens, there are several things to keep in mind. You must:

1. Take enough vitamin C
2. Take it frequently, to keep blood levels high

3. Take it for long enough, don't stop taking it until you are well

The most common types of vitamin C:

1. Ascorbic acid
2. Liposomal
3. Sodium ascorbate
4. Calcium ascorbate

Ascorbic Acid

Ascorbic acid is the chemical name for vitamin C. Since vitamin C is so acidic, it is often buffered to reduce acidity. It can be combined with sodium, calcium, magnesium, potassium, and other minerals. Once it is combined with these other minerals, the vitamin C name changes from ascorbic acid to sodium ascorbate, calcium ascorbate, magnesium ascorbate, and potassium ascorbate.

Sodium Ascorbate

Vitamin C is buffered by sodium. The type of sodium used is not the type that causes fluid retention.

Calcium Ascorbate

Ascorbic acid buffered with calcium is called calcium ascorbate. High doses of calcium taken without the opposing magnesium are discouraged by most vitamin C experts. Each product has different amounts of calcium per serving, so you will need to check the label.

Unless the calcium is combined with magnesium, or only a very small amount of calcium is used, I would not prefer to take that product. One brand I found contained 500 mg. of calcium per four grams of vitamin C. It also had no magnesium to balance the calcium.

Dosage

Most vitamin C advocates suggest everyone take 5,000 mg. per day. This is 5 grams, which can be done easily with most powdered supplements, with a teaspoon daily.

Liposomal Vitamin C

Although in an ideal world, IV vitamin C would be available to everyone to treat infections, it is not. There seems to be little interest in the medical establishment to help people with it.

Since we need to help ourselves, we need options. Liposomal vitamin C is considered to be as effective as IV vitamin C.

Vitamin C is processed with phosphatidylcholine (PC). This is a type of lipid, or fat. Processing vitamin C like this enables it to be better absorbed. This helps it to bypass stomach acid. Your body will allow more liposomal C to be absorbed at one time.

I have had great results with Lypo-Spheric liposomal vitamin C by LivOn Labs. I have not used any of the other brands that have recently started making liposomal C.

Intravenous Vitamin C

Intravenous vitamin C is the best option, if it is available to you. Vitamin C is usually administered as sodium ascorbate, which is absorbed very well. Dr. Frederick R. Klenner, MD, wrote a book called *Clinical Guide to the Use of Vitamin C*. He details how he used IV vitamin C to cure many diseases. This book is out of print, but available for free online as a PDF.

Combine Antiviral Herbs with Vitamin C

I did not fully understand how potent vitamin C is to resolve infections. I have always depended on herbal medicine to treat viruses, and I get great results. What I found is that herbs are amazing to treat viruses, but when combined with high dosages of vitamin C, it is virtually unbelievable how fast you can get better.

I also found that the vitamin C energized me, and it cleared my brain. Your brain has a higher need for vitamin C than the rest of your body.

Most people have heard that vitamin C will help the immune system to resolve a cold. What surprised me the most when doing research for this book is that so much research has already been done that confirms the effectiveness of vitamin C to treat viruses and bacteria.

The problem is that if you are already in a hospital with a serious infection, you will probably not be able to get intravenous C, because there are no protocols in place for that. Once you are in the hospital, it is too late!

If I had an infection, I would take Chinese herbal medicine, and one gram of vitamin C every hour. This can be easily done using capsules.

Liposomal vitamin C is three to four times as effective as regular vitamin C supplements.

Research:

Carr AC, Rowe S. The Emerging Role of Vitamin C in the Prevention and Treatment of COVID-19. Nutrients. 2020 Oct 27;12(11):3286. doi:

10.3390/nu12113286. PMID: 33121019; PMCID: PMC7693980.

Medical doctors as of the date of this writing do not use intravenous vitamin C to treat Covid, or any other infection in most hospitals. It is not even easy to find a vitamin infusion center that will use high enough doses of vitamin C infusions to help people.

There is always the risk that someone will complain about the service provided, and the medical doctor could lose his or her license for practicing medicine outside of the established medical norms. A doctor who does this could lose the ability to practice medicine, and lose his or her livelihood after many years of hard work. I believe that change will have to be made from the bottom up. People will have to demand their family members get vitamin C infusions if they are in the hospital.

Hidden Viruses Cause Disease

Many people have viruses lurking in their bodies and do not know it. The most common symptom is fatigue. It is worthwhile to take higher doses of vitamin C for a while and see if this helps relieve your fatigue.

Viruses and bacteria are a part of our lives. We cannot kill them all. Most of them are not harmful, but your immune system needs enough vitamin C to protect you from the ones that are harmful.

Vitamin C Books

Dr. Thomas E. Levy is a vitamin C expert. He has been at the forefront of research and spreading the word about what vitamin C heals for many years. I'm sure he has had to face ridicule from other medical doctors about his claims to cure disease with vitamin C, but he has not let that stop him.

Dr. Levy has written numerous books and articles on vitamin C detailing how vitamin C has been used to treat diseases, and how to use it in a hospital setting.

He has written extensively about liposomal vitamin C and how it can often replace IV vitamin C. Since we usually will not be able to get IV vitamin C at all, it is good to know there is a substitute.

For further research on vitamin C, and the many diseases it can treat, you can read Dr. Levy's books. A few titles are: *Curing the Incurable, Primal Panacea, Stop America's #1 Killer,* and

Rapid Virus Recovery. His website is at www.peakenergy.com.

A few diseases detailed in his books which have been shown to be treatable with vitamin C at high doses are:

- Polio
- Pneumonia
- Mumps
- Mononucleosis
- Tuberculosis
- Dementia/Alzheimer's
- Encephalitis
- Measles

Can Vitamin C Clean Out Arteries? (atherosclerosis)

If you would like to prevent the likelihood of heart attacks and strokes, taking a simple supplement might help you.

Linus Pauling was a two-time Nobel prize winning scientist. He became an advocate of using vitamin C. His theory is that a lack of vitamin C is what causes your body to form plaque inside of your arteries. When you are vitamin C deficient, your body has to patch up your arteries to keep you alive.

Scurvy is caused by a lack of vitamin C. This disease causes the blood vessels to leak, because collagen cannot be made by the body without enough vitamin C. By taking vitamin C, lysine, and proline, your body is able to dissolve the fatty plaque.

I know this sounds nuts. But I simply cannot talk about vitamin C without giving you this information. There are many products combining vitamin C, lysine, and proline. Heart Plus from Cell Nutritionals is a good one. Please refer to the *book Stop America's #1 Killer*, by Dr. Levy. This book explains how to treat and prevent heart disease with supplements.

Vitamin C Dosage for Serious Infections

Your body can quickly use up your vitamin C stores when you are sick. Vitamin C is water soluble, and your body does not store a lot.

One way to determine how much vitamin C you need is to take high doses until you get loose stools. Your body will consume high amounts of vitamin C when you are sick.

If you take liposomal vitamin C, it is unlikely you will get loose stools. It is absorbed very well, which means your effective dosage can be much lower.

If you take ascorbic acid powder, take 10 grams, which should be about two teaspoons. If you do not have loose stools, take another 10 grams. Keep repeating until you get water stools.

According to Dr. Sarah Myhill, most people need 3-4 doses to abolish symptoms. This would be 30 to 40 grams per day. She also suggests a low carb diet, because viruses and bacteria feed on sugar, and multiply faster.

Even if your symptoms are gone, that does not mean the virus is completely gone, so it would be a good idea to continue taking vitamin C like this for five days or so. There is no reason not to.

8

Vitamin C Powders and Product Reviews

Vitamin C is most effective if it is taken in high enough doses, and as frequently as possible. It is easy and inexpensive to take the powder form, but there are several different types to consider.

I tested several brands for this book. I wanted to compare the solubility, and taste of these products, to give you a comparison.

Ascorbic acid is basic vitamin C, that is the most common type sold. But it is very sour. When ascorbic acid is buffered with sodium, it become sodium ascorbate, and that is salty.

Dosage Size

If I had an active infection, I would try to get 1,000 mg. every hour, or every other hour. Taking it throughout the day will help maintain higher blood levels, because it is water soluble, and it will not build up in your system. Your body uses up vitamin C quickly when you are sick. The only downside to taking too much, is loose stools. That only happens if your body does not absorb everything you consumed.

For maintenance, I think one Lypospheric vitamin C per day from LivOn labs is great.

There is some disagreement on whether the amount of calcium used in calcium ascorbate is too much. It is not recommended to take high doses of calcium every day, long term. Each brand is formulated with differing amounts of calcium.

Hard Water vs. Soft Water

When I first started testing vitamin C powder, I found it hard to dissolve. If I could get it to dissolve at all, it took a long time. I tried using boiling water, that worked, but then I found out that you cannot use boiling water on vitamin C, because it destroys it.

I found that combining it with a small amount of honey did work, but I knew that was a bad idea, as the sugar in the honey might be too much, and affect the absorption of the vitamin C.

Then it occurred to me that perhaps it was my water. I use reverse osmosis water. The filtering process pulls the minerals out. I then tested the vitamin C powders in tap water and they dissolved with no problem.

If you live in a soft water area, or use filtered water, be aware it might be more difficult to dissolve your vitamin C powder.

C-Salts, from Wholesale Nutrition

My first choice for vitamin C powder is C-Salts. This product is made by Wholesale Nutrition. It is buffered with calcium, magnesium, zinc, and potassium. It fizzes when you add water to it.

In one teaspoon you get 4 grams of vitamin C, buffered with calcium at 145 mg., magnesium at 55 mg., and zinc at 2 mg. It also has 365 mg. of potassium. A teaspoon contains 14% of your daily requirement of these minerals, so it is not enough, but it is a start. Their website is www.nutri.com.

Supplement Facts
Serving size: One teaspoon (5.27 gr)

Amount per Teaspoon		% Daily Value*
Vitamin C (as 1-Ascorbate)	4000 mg	6700%
Calcium (as Ascorbate)	145 mg	14%
Magnesium (as Ascorbate)	55 mg	14%
Zinc (as Ascorbate)	2 mg	14%
Potassium (as Ascorbate)	365 mg	**14%

*Percent of U.S. RDA for adults.
**RDA not established. This is a research estimate.

Some brands of buffered ascorbic acid contain higher amounts of calcium. One brand I found had 610 mg. of calcium, for 5,000 mg. of ascorbic acid. That will make the vitamin C less sour, but it also does not have magnesium to balance out the calcium.

Many people are deficient in potassium, and they don't know it. It can cause muscle cramps, and muscle weakness. The daily minimum requirement of potassium is 4,700 mg. according to most sources.

Calcium and Magnesium

Some vitamin C experts prefer pure ascorbic acid over buffered vitamin C. Although calcium should be taken with magnesium, and I do not recommend taking calcium by itself, many people are deficient in calcium and magnesium. This causes many ailments, and it seems to me that this supplement covers its bases by adding magnesium.

Phosphoric Acid Can Damage Bones

Soft drinks have phosphoric acid in them. Even one drink can deplete your calcium levels to a serious degree. Your body uses calcium to buffer the acid in soft drinks. In my experience, it can cause bone pain if you drink soft drinks regularly.

It is very hard to consume enough calcium which your body needs to buffer acid. If you do not get enough calcium, your body can pull this from your bones. This can deplete your bones over time.

There are supplements that can help you restore your bones. I like Raw Calcium, by Garden of Life, which has calcium, magnesium and other bone growth co-factors in it. It is very well absorbed. Calcium should not be taken as a single supplement. Ever. I know those chocolate chews with just calcium carbonate in them are tempting, but calcium carbonate is not well absorbed anyway.

One of my uncles has diabetic neuropathy. He took calcium supplements and it reduced his pain somewhat. If you are deficient in vitamins or minerals, it can easily cause deficiency diseases.

Potassium

Per serving size of 3.5 oz., a banana contains about 358 mg. of potassium, raw spinach is 558 mg., and tomato paste is 1,014 mg.

According to www.nutritionfacts.org:

"Less than 2% of Americans even get the recommended minimum adequate intake of 4,700 a day. To get even the adequate intake, the average American would have to eat like 5 more bananas worth of potassium a day. 98% of Americans eat potassium deficient diets because they don't eat enough plants.

Why do we care? A review of all the best studies ever done on potassium intake and its relationship to two of our top killers, stroke and heart disease, was recently published in the *Journal of the American College of Cardiology*.

A 1,600mg per day higher potassium intake was associated with a 21% lower risk of stroke. That still wouldn't get the average American up to the minimum adequate intake, but it might be able to wipe out a fifth of their stroke risk. The paper concludes: "These results support recommendations for higher consumption of potassium-rich foods to prevent vascular diseases."

Potassium citrate is available in powder form, as a supplement. I have seen potassium supplements relieve muscle cramps, and tight, weak muscles. Potassium capsules or tablets are regulated by the government to contain only 100 mg. potassium. This would require you to take 470 tablets for your daily minimum dose.

Doctor's Best Pure Vitamin C Powder, Quali-C

I felt this was good quality ascorbic acid, and it is made in Scotland. It comes with a little scoop, which measures one gram.

NutriBiotic Sodium Ascorbate

This product is one of my favorite powders. One of the things that stood out the most is that they had capsules with more vitamin C in them was the capsule size. If you would like to take capsules, NutriBiotic makes capsules that have 850 mg. vitamin C each. They are about the same size as other companies encapsulated 500 mg. vitamin C, which means they have no added fillers. A lot of people do not like to take large tablets or capsules, so this size issue is important to note.

An alternative to taking powders during an acute viral infection is to take two 500 mg capsules or tablets per hour. Do whatever makes you feel most comfortable.

Long before I knew about the antiviral effect of high doses of vitamin C, I took Chinese herbs, which helped me prevent a full blown cold or flu. Vitamin C is not completely necessary, but it will help you get better a lot faster.

9

Curcumin Antiviral Benefits and Product Reviews

There is a lot of research on curcumin. It is not classically used as an antiviral. In Chinese medicine it is used to treat inflammation and pain. It is not used as a single herb, it is combined with other herbs in formulas. Since I believe this might help people prevent viral infections, I wanted to give it its own chapter.

I was a little disturbed by some of the marketing claims being made by some supplement companies about their curcumin. As an herbalist, I get upset when I think people are being misled or ripped off when buying supplements. So, I bought a bunch of curcumin supplements and did research and testing on the products. This will hopefully help you save money, and get a quality product.

Antiviral and Wonder Herb

Curcumin has unexpected antiviral properties. Once I started looking for references for the antiviral aspect of this herb, I uncovered a lot of other exciting information. So, I hope you don't mind that I included this research. In addition to the antiviral effects, I was excited to know that it has a rejuvenating effect on the brain, and it treats cognitive issues.

Curcumin or Turmeric

The common name of this herb is turmeric, and the Latin name is curcuma longa. Curcuminoids are regularly referred to as the most important part of turmeric, so that is probably why both names are used.

Curcumin is very popular to treat inflammation and pain. It can be taken daily for extended periods of time. It can make the blood less likely to clot, so if you are taking blood thinners, make sure you speak with your healthcare provider about taking this. Please refer to the blood clot prevention chapter for information on clotting.

Turmeric Benefits

Turmeric:

- Relieves inflammation
- Thins the blood
- Treats liver and gallbladder issues
- Treats fatty liver
- Relieves pain
- Has antiviral benefits

As with most herbs, an herbal extract is the best choice. Curcumin has a very pungent smell. If you open a bottle of curcumin, and do not smell anything, or just a faint smell, it might not be an effective supplement.

Preventing Viral Infections

Research suggests curcumin might be helpful to prevent a viral infection. It is reported to inhibit SARS and Covid viruses by multiple mechanisms: direct interaction with viral membrane proteins, disruption of the viral envelope, inhibition of viral proteases.

Research:

Thimmulappa RK, Mudnakudu-Nagaraju KK, Shivamallu C, Subramaniam KJT, Radhakrishnan A, Bhojraj S, Kuppusamy G. Antiviral and immunomodulatory activity of curcumin: A case for prophylactic therapy for COVID-19. Heliyon. 2021 Feb;7(2):e06350. doi: 10.1016/j.heliyon.2021.e06350. Epub 2021 Feb 22. PMID: 33655086; PMCID: PMC7899028.

Buying Quality Curcumin/Turmeric

Curcumin is considered to be hard to absorb, so it is often combined with a small amount of piperine, which is pepper.

Curcumin and Lecithin

Curcumin is absorbed better if it is combined with Lecithin. Lecithin is a type of fat, it can be used to treat fatty liver, and improve brain function. It is also called phosphatidylcholine. It is an emulsifier of fat. It breaks down fat kind of like detergent breaks down fat.

Indian food cooks are experts at cooking with strong spices. They often mix their spices with a small amount of oil, and heat it a little before adding them to food. I believe combining or processing curcumin with lecithin, uses the same theory.

Research about lecithin and curcumin:

> Peng S, Zou L, Liu W, Liu C, McClements DJ. Fabrication and Characterization of Curcumin-Loaded Liposomes Formed from Sunflower Lecithin: Impact of Composition and Environmental Stress. J Agric Food Chem. 2018 Nov 21;66(46):12421-12430. doi: 10.1021/acs.jafc.8b04136. Epub 2018 Nov 8. PMID: 30372060.

Curcumin Products Reviewed

The short answer to which brands I believe are the best option, is Nature's Way, and Planetary Herbals. These are both tablets and when you open the bottle, you smell how aromatic they are.

Planetary Herbals is called Full Spectrum Turmeric Extract. It also has a slightly sweet smell, but it is very pleasant smelling. Nature's Way is called Turmeric Premium Extract. Both of these products smell very pleasant.

There were two brands that surprised me. I normally love these brands, but I believe their products were not as strong as the other brands I tried. When I test an herb, and it has no smell, it is usually not a good sign. Strong herbs are aromatic. The two companies are Jarrow, and Doctor's Best. I even taste tested the Doctor's Best turmeric. There was no taste at all. I had an old bottle of Nature's Way curcumin, and it still had a nice aromatic smell. So, I don't think the age of the herb was a factor.

Some of the curcumin products I tested smelled rancid. I will not name brand names, but I will include the ingredients. One brand listed acacia gum, rice hull concentrate, rice hulls, organic Arabic, and other ingredients. I believe they used too much oil in this product, and it has spoiled. Rancid oil is very unhealthy to consume, it can damage your cells.

Another brand contains what they called essential oils of turmeric. It also smells rancid. Essential oils can spoil if heated, or exposed to oxygen for too long. Any supplement that smells rotten is probably oxidized. Products with oil in them have to be carefully preserved with antioxidants, to prevent spoilage.

Yet another product had a high percentage of fenugreek. It is believed that this enhances the absorption of the curcumin. I thought it smelled very unpleasant.

Another type of curcumin product is fermented turmeric. They ferment turmeric with acidophilus. They claim it has a higher percentage of curcumin, and that it is better absorbed. Since this product is so new, it is hard to compare it to traditionally processed turmeric. Other than a few articles, curcumin research has been done on traditionally processed turmeric. Personally, I would pass on this, until I have more information.

The best way to determine which product works best for you is to try several brands. Some people get great results with some of the products that I did not personally like.

Curcumin Marketing Claims

Curcumin products are big business these days. There are some companies that are charging three times as much for their products as the brands I listed. Some claim they have a proprietary product. They claim that their product has more of the active ingredient in curcumin. A lot of the claims being made are not supportable, and they seem to be marketing claims.

Curcumin Helps your Brain

Curcumin has been tested and found to be effective in preventing the accumulation of Beta Amyloid in the brain. Research shows curcumin has the following brain functions:

- Anti-inflammatory
- Anti-arthritis
- Boosts memory and cognitive function
- Crosses the blood-brain barrier, to reach brain cells
- Protects neurons from various toxic insults of aging and Beta amyloid
- Relieves cognitive decline
- Improves synaptic functions

Research:

Reddy PH, Manczak M, Yin X, Grady MC, Mitchell A, Tonk S, Kuruva CS, Bhatti JS, Kandimalla R, Vijayan M, Kumar S, Wang R, Pradeepkiran JA, Ogunmokun G, Thamarai K, Quesada K, Boles A, Reddy AP. Protective Effects of Indian Spice Curcumin Against Amyloid-β in Alzheimer's Disease. J Alzheimers Dis. 2018;61(3):843-866. doi:

10.3233/JAD-170512. PMID: 29332042; PMCID: PMC5796761.

Beta amyloid protein is the tissue in the brain that is involved with Alzheimer's and cognitive decline. It is not known if the Beta amyloid causes Alzheimer's or if something else causes the Beta amyloid, which leads to Alzheimer's symptoms.

Of course, curcumin is antiviral, and there is research indicating that dementia can be caused by infections.

Another research article states that curcumin-loaded nanoparticles potently induce adult neurogenesis and reverse cognitive deficits in Alzheimer's disease model.

Curcumin:

- Induces new brain cell growth by targeting neural stem cells
- Improves the brain's self-regenerative capacity
- Protects the brain from damage
- Reverses learning and memory impairments in an amyloid beta induced rat model of Alzheimer's-like phenotypes
- Enhance the brain's self-repair mechanism.

Research:

Tiwari SK, Agarwal S, Seth B, Yadav A, Nair S, Bhatnagar P, Karmakar M, Kumari M, Chauhan LK, Patel DK, Srivastava V, Singh D, Gupta SK, Tripathi A, Chaturvedi RK, Gupta KC. Curcumin-loaded nanoparticles potently induce adult neurogenesis and reverse cognitive deficits in Alzheimer's disease model via canonical Wnt/β-catenin pathway. ACS Nano. 2014 Jan 28;8(1):76-103. doi: 10.1021/nn405077y. Epub 2013 Dec 10. Erratum in: ACS Nano. 2019 Jun 25;13(6):7355. PMID: 24467380.

Research Dosage for Antiviral Benefits

It is difficult to know how much curcumin to take to get the antiviral benefits. Each study is done with a different type of curcumin, and some of them use an isolated compound, not the whole herb.

The following study used a very low dosage, but still showed very good results. The dosage used was 80 mg. twice a day. That is a pretty low dosage of an herb. This might indicate how strong curcumin is, if a dose that low is effective. Most herbs would be taken two to three times daily.

The article says that curcumin inhibits the virus entrance into the cell, the encapsulation and replication, and modulated various cellular signaling pathways. The duration of treatment for COVID-19 patients was "meaningfully shorter."

Further, “no patient in treatment group experienced deterioration of infection during follow-up period, but it occurred in 40% of control group. “

They also reported that curcumin had a direct and indirect antiviral activity against HIV by inhibiting virus replication or via blocking inflammatory pathways operating in the acquired immunodeficiency syndrome. The HIV research was by Prasad & Tyagi, 2015.

HIV Research:

Prasad S, Tyagi AK. Curcumin and its analogues: a potential natural compound against HIV infection and AIDS. Food Funct. 2015 Nov;6(11):3412-9. doi: 10.1039/c5fo00485c. Epub 2015 Sep 25. PMID: 26404185.

COVID-19 Research:

Saber-Moghaddam N, Salari S, Hejazi S, Amini M, Taherzadeh Z, Eslami S, Rezayat SM, Jaafari MR, Elyasi S. Oral nano-curcumin formulation efficacy in management of mild to moderate hospitalized coronavirus disease-19 patients: An open label nonrandomized clinical trial. Phytother Res. 2021 Jan 3. doi: 10.1002/ptr.7004. Epub ahead of print. PMID: 33389761.

Until I have a personal experience with curcumin knocking out a viral infection, I will continue to recommend Chinese herbs. However, I am intrigued by the amount of research that is being done on curcumin, and how it has been tested against AIDS. I would tend to take it to prevent a cold, rather than treat an active infection. Perhaps taking it regularly will prevent a virus infection from starting in the first place.

I would not recommend curcumin for people on blood thinners. It is in the blood thinning category. This would also mean care should be taken on both dosage and length of time taken. Lower doses are less likely to cause side effects.

10

Cordyceps Benefits and Product Reviews

Cordyceps is a fungus that is one of the strongest herbal tonics available. It is one of the best herbs to treat fatigue. It can also be used daily to boost the immune system. It can also be combined with other antiviral herbs. If you have a weak immune system, it is very important to take tonic herbs like cordyceps to strengthen it.

Cordyceps, Dong Chong Xia Cao, Cordyceps sinensis

Cordyceps is not a standard part of Chinese herbal medicine, because it has traditionally been very expensive. However, it is increasingly being used and added to herbal tonics, which are used to improve energy, and overall health. It works by strengthening the kidneys, lungs, and heart, which will treat hundreds of diseases.

Cordyceps:

- Strengthens the kidneys, which treats fatigue, frequent urination, impotence, premature ejaculation, tinnitus, and memory issues.

- Strengthens the lungs, which treats coughing, caused by weak lungs as in asthma, or excess mucus production from any cause.
- Treats allergies by strengthening the lungs.
- Treats tinnitus, which is caused by weak kidneys in Chinese medicine.

This herb is not in the clear toxic heat category, so it is not considered to treat viral infections, but modern research indicates that it actually is antiviral. I sometimes combine it with antiviral herbs.

Antiviral herbs treat the virus, but your immune system still has to be strong enough to fight off the viruses that have already multiplied in your body. Cordyceps is a wonderful immune tonic.

There are different parts of the cordyceps fungus. The fruiting body is the strongest part. The mycelium is the little roots attached to the fruiting body. They do have some activity, but they are not usually the best option.

Mycelium vs. Fruiting Body

Some supplement manufacturers use the mycelium, because it is much less expensive. The fruiting body extract is the best choice. Good quality cordyceps has a nice nutty smell to it. It is usually a darker tan color.

Freshcap mushrooms makes a good cordyceps fruiting body extract powder. Real Mushrooms and Freshcap are two products I have found to be good quality. Cordyceps can be cultured on different mediums, giving it a different smell and flavor. Some companies culture it on tree bark.

The Real Mushrooms brand, and Freshcap brand are both good options. This herb is one of the most potent herbs to boost energy levels, so take it with breakfast and lunch if you are taking it to prevent a viral infection.

Cordyceps Militaris vs. Sinensis

Cordyceps sinensis is the traditional type of cordyceps, used as an expensive tonic for years. It appears that this type of cordyceps is very expensive now, and hard to cultivate. This means that if you want to take the fruiting body extract, you will need to take cordyceps militaris.

Cordyceps Research

Cordyceps is believed to be effective in controlling SARS-CoV-2 replication. Cordycepin, a component in cordyceps, has anti-viral activity against several viruses including influenza, human immunodeficiency virus, murine leukemia virus, plant viruses, and Epstein-Barr virus.

Research:

Ohta Y, Lee JB, Hayashi K, Fujita A, Park DK, Hayashi T. In vivo anti-influenza virus activity of an immunomodulatory acidic polysaccharide isolated from Cordyceps militaris grown on germinated soybeans. J Agric Food Chem. 2007 Dec 12;55(25):10194-9. doi: 10.1021/jf0721287. Epub 2007 Nov 8. PMID: 17988090.

Cordyceps extracts inhibit viral replication.

Research:

Verma AK. Cordycepin: a bioactive metabolite of *Cordyceps militaris* and polyadenylation inhibitor with therapeutic potential against COVID-19. J Biomol Struct Dyn. 2020 Nov 23:1-8. doi: 10.1080/07391102.2020.1850352. Epub ahead of print. PMID: 33225826; PMCID: PMC7754931.

This quote is interesting. The cordycepin is just one compound in cordyceps. Using the complete, whole herb is how things are done in Chinese medicine. Scientists like to isolate compounds in herbs, and test for one specific part. But it is saying that cordyceps stops the influenza viruses from reproducing, which would mean it is much harder for a virus to cause a serious infection.

Asthma

One of my patients had asthma her entire life, which in Chinese medicine is caused by weak lungs. She was able to recover from that by taking cordyceps for an extended period of time. It is very helpful to take tonic herbs. They improve health and longevity.

One research article concluded that cordyceps sinensis improved asthma symptoms, lung function, and inflammatory profile of the patients with moderate to severe asthma.

Research:

Wang N, Li J, Huang X, Chen W, Chen Y. Herbal Medicine *Cordyceps sinensis* Improves Health-Related Quality of Life in Moderate-to-Severe Asthma. Evid Based Complement Alternat Med. 2016;2016:6134593. doi: 10.1155/2016/6134593. Epub 2016 Dec 5. PMID: 28050193; PMCID: PMC5165155.

Fatigue

The following research article concludes that cordyceps militaris “significantly delayed fatigue phenomenon”, increased ATP levels and antioxidative enzymes activity, and reduced the levels of lactic acid. They state that "When fatigue happens, it will gradually accumulate and eventually lead to overstrain, endocrine disorders, a weakened immune system, even organ lesions."

Research:

Song J, Wang Y, Teng M, Cai G, Xu H, Guo H, Liu Y, Wang D, Teng L. Studies on the Antifatigue Activities of Cordyceps militaris Fruit Body Extract in Mouse Model. Evid Based Complement Alternat Med. 2015;2015:174616. doi: 10.1155/2015/174616. Epub 2015 Aug 17. PMID: 26351509; PMCID: PMC4553310.

My preferred brands for cordyceps fruiting body are Real Mushrooms, and Freshcap Mushrooms. They also make combine several mushrooms in one product, which will give you the benefit of all of them in one product. Mushrooms are taken to boost the immune system.

The Real Mushroom Brand formula is called 5 Defenders. Freshcap is called Thrive 6. I would consider both of these products. They also have very informative websites if you would like to do further research on mushrooms. Real Mushrooms is at www.realmushrooms.com. Freshcap is at www.freshcap.com.

In doing research for this article, I came across information stating that most cordyceps sinensis on the market is not the fruiting body. This news will be upsetting for people who thought they were using the cordyceps sinensis fruiting body extract. It upset me anyway.

The Real Mushroom company has extensive information on this. They culture their own mushrooms.

> The following is copied from the Real Mushrooms website:
>
> Types of Cordyceps Supplements
> There are 3 types of Cordyceps supplements that are commonly found on the market as replacements for the extravagantly-priced *Cordyceps sinensis*:
> Cordyceps CS-4
> Cordyceps Myceliated Grain
> Extract of Cordyceps Mushrooms (Militaris)
> Cordyceps Cs-4
>
> In the 1980s, when wild *Cordyceps sinensis* was gaining in popularity and the price tag kept climbing, scientists in China set out to cultivate this fungus. Many tried and many failed. Still to this day, there is **no affordable** cultivated version of this mushroom. What the scientists did end up with are Cordyceps anamorphs, mycelium cultures that are unable to produce a mushroom (fruiting body).
> These anamorphs were grown in a liquid growth medium to create mass amounts of pure mycelium.

This process is known as liquid culture mycelium, or liquid fermentation, and involves **growing the mycelium in a liquid solution of nutrients that can then be removed, leaving you with pure mycelium.** Most mycelium research is based on liquid fermentation mycelium.

These anamorphs were studied extensively and found to produce similar results to wild *Cordyceps sinensis*. This ended up turning into what is now known as **Cordyceps Cs-4.** After undergoing clinical trials in China, the Chinese government approved its use in TCM (Traditional Chinese Medicine) hospitals and it is now recognized as a safe natural product in China.

If a Cordyceps supplement is claiming to be *Cordyceps sinensis* and it is made in China, it is almost certainly Cordyceps Cs-4.
Other Cs-4 products may also be labeled as *Paecilomyces hepiali*, which is an anamorph form of *Cordyceps sinensis*.

Do not confuse Cordyceps Cs-4 (pure mycelium) with Cordyceps myceliated grain (below), as these are very different products.

https://www.realmushrooms.com/cordyceps-supplements-guide/#772ph

I would prefer to take the cordyceps militaris fruiting body extract, over the cordyceps sinensis mycelium.

11

Blood Clot Prevention and Treatment

The reason I am including information about blood clotting and thick blood is that some viruses, like COVID-19, can cause blood clotting disorders. In fact, this is considered to be one of the most serious aspects of this virus.

Most herbs regulate the blood, which reduces clotting. They make it less likely the blood will clot. So, if you are on blood thinners, you will definitely want to consult your health care provider to make sure the herbs in this category are OK for you. Acupuncturists with herbal training will also be able to work with you on this. Although enzymes are usually a better option for most people.

COVID-19 Clots

One of the things that has made COVID-19 so devastating is blood clots. According to reports, even people who are taking blood thinning drugs are still getting clots when they have this virus.

According to one study from the Netherlands, 31% of patients hospitalized with Covid got clots while on blood thinners. Notice that they were already taking drugs to thin their blood, but they got blood clots anyway.

Research:

Klok, F A et al. "Incidence of thrombotic complications in critically ill ICU patients with COVID-19." *Thrombosis research* vol. 191 (2020): 145-147. doi:10.1016/j.thromres. 2020.04.013

Blood clots can easily cause heart attacks, and stroke, as well as pulmonary embolisms. The blood clot can go anywhere in your body and block blood flow, or oxygen flow, and can be deadly.

Blood Stasis is Thick Blood

Chinese herbal medicine has been used to treat blood clots for thousands of years. It is a very important part of pain relief. If there is a lack of healthy circulation, the blood can pool in that area, it is called Blood Stasis.

Blood stasis can be mild, and easily resolved, or the blood thickness can be very serious. As we age, we tend to have thicker blood. When we are less active, our blood is also thicker, and does not circulate as well.

Any time the blood is too thick, it can cause pain. That is why so many of the herbs in this chapter can also relieve pain. The enzymes also are amazing to treat pain, and prevent blood clots.

Always Treat the Virus

Regardless of symptoms, the since the cause of the symptoms is a virus, the virus must be treated. Treat it as soon as you think you have an infection. Treat it early and often.

Curcumin as a Blood Thinner

Please refer to the chapter on curcumin for details on brands. Curcumin is included in this chapter, because it is a blood thinning herb.

Research on Curcumin and blood clots:

Suresh P. S. (2020). Curcumin and Coagulopathy in the COVID19 Era. *Indian journal of clinical biochemistry : IJCB*, *35*(4), 1–2. Advance online publication. https://doi.org/10.1007/s12291-020-00914-5

This report discusses how curcumin and bromelain (pineapple enzyme) can be used to reduce clotting.

Research:

Kritis P, Karampela I, Kokoris S, Dalamaga M. The combination of bromelain and curcumin as an immune-boosting nutraceutical in the prevention of severe COVID-19. Metabol Open. 2020 Dec;8:100066. doi: 10.1016/j.metop.2020.100066. Epub 2020 Nov 13. PMID: 33205039; PMCID: PMC7661945.

Here is a study on how curcumin can be used to treat deep vein thrombosis.

Research:

Wang T, Guan R, Xia F, Du J, Xu L. Curcumin promotes venous thrombi resolve process in a mouse deep venous thrombosis model via regulating miR-499. Microvasc Res. 2021 Jul;136:104148. doi: 10.1016/j.mvr.2021.104148. Epub 2021 Feb 23. PMID: 33631181.

Many people suffer from blood clots in the legs. Taking curcumin regularly could help prevent this. Thick blood is often common in older people, that is one reason they suffer from pain more often.

Boswellin

Boswellin is also called frankincense. It is called Ru Xiang in Chinese. This herb is much stronger than curcumin. I would not take this herb long term. This herb is not used as a single herb in Chinese medicine, it is used in combination with other herbs in formulas. It is also used in topical pain relief formulas, because it helps to move the blood, improve circulation to relieve pain.

Boswellin relieves blood stasis, relieves pain, and swelling. It is bitter and warm. You might recognize that frankincense and myrrh were mentioned in the bible. That is how long these herbs have been used. At least 2,000 years.

Boswellin research, they use the term Boswellic Acid:

Wang M, Chen M, Ding Y, Zhu Z, Zhang Y, Wei P, Wang J, Qiao Y, Li L, Li Y, Wen A. Pretreatment with β-Boswellic Acid Improves Blood Stasis Induced Endothelial Dysfunction: Role of eNOS Activation. Sci Rep. 2015 Oct 20;5:15357. doi: 10.1038/srep15357. PMID: 26482008; PMCID: PMC4611516.

Proteolytic Enzymes Can Dissolve Blood Clots

Enzymes are very effective to relieve pain, inflammation, and to prevent and resolve blood clots. There are different types of enzymes. Each type of enzyme only dissolves the thing it was made to dissolve.

The most commonly used enzyme to dissolve blood clots is protease. Enzymes dissolve protein and fibrin. They can break down extra tissue in your bloodstream, as well as scar tissue. All the enzymes in this chapter are proteases.

- Protease enzymes dissolve protein
- Amylase enzymes dissolve starch
- Lipase enzymes dissolve fat
- Cellulase enzymes dissolve fiber

Enzymes for Digestion and Cellular Repair

Your body makes its own enzymes. These enzymes are used to digest your food. They are also used to repair damaged tissue. Once the damaged tissue has been broken down, healthy tissue can be formed.

Aging and Enzymes

As we age, our body is not able to make as many enzymes as it did when we were younger. This is why we are more likely to have thick blood, and blood clots. That is why so many people take pharmaceutical blood thinners when they get to a certain age. Blood thinners help to reduce the likelihood of blood clots which can lead to heart attacks and strokes.

Taking enzymes with your meals will help you digest your meal, which might improve your energy levels. But there will be fewer enzymes available to circulate in your body for cellular repair.

Enzymes taken between meals, go into your bloodstream and your body uses them for cellular repair. They treat inflammation, scar tissue, and thick blood.

Bromelain

Bromelain is a protease enzyme derived from pineapples. Canned pineapple has to be boiled to kill bacteria, so the enzymes are destroyed. Enzymes are very sensitive to heat and humidity, and are definitely destroyed when boiled.

Some people think they are allergic to pineapple, because when they eat it, they get a sore tongue. The reason they have a sore tongue is that the bromelain enzyme dissolves the coating on the tongue, and if you eat a lot of it, it can irritate your tongue or any tissue inside your mouth.

Raw pineapple is a source of bromelain, or you can take supplements. Bromelain is very effective to treat inflammation and pain. If you take a bromelain pill a half hour before breakfast, or any meal, you will find inflammation will be greatly relieved if not resolved completely.

2,000 Active Units Minimum Per Pill

Enzymes are measured in active units, not milligrams. So, 500 milligrams from one supplement company might have more active units than one from another. I prefer to use at least 2,000 GDU at a time. With that strength you can get often get pain relief with one pill.

If I were taking bromelain to thin the blood, I would take 2,000 GDU units twice a day. Be careful with your dosage. If the dosage is too high, it could irritate the stomach lining. The bromelain can dissolve the mucus lining in your stomach and irritate the stomach walls.

Taking enzymes on an empty stomach usually prevents stomach issues, which are rare, but possible. The enzymes do not remain in the stomach a long time when it is empty. They quickly travel to the small intestine, where they are absorbed.

As a natural anti-inflammatory and anticoagulant, bromelain is being considered as a COVID-19 supplement. Proteases have been used for years to help the body fight viruses. I would not depend on this as my first choice to fight viruses, but it treats many aspects of viruses that cause blood clots and severe inflammation. It does this naturally, with no side effects.

Enzymes are much stronger than pharmaceuticals, because they actually dissolve the blood clot. From what I understand, pharmaceutical blood thinners work by reducing the production of clotting factors. One product was described as 'blocking the platelets from sticking together." I think each drug works in a different way, but I don't think most of them actually dissolve blood clots. They inhibit platelet aggregation, which means the blood platelets are less likely to stick together. Ginger root does this also. It is not used to break down blood clots, but it does inhibit platelet aggregation. The enzymes work on dead tissue only, from what I understand.

Research:

Owoyele BV, Bakare AO, Ologe MO. Bromelain: A Review on its Potential as a Therapy for the Management of Covid-19. Niger J Physiol Sci. 2020 Jun 30;35(1):10-19. PMID: 33084621.

Research on ginger and platelet aggregation:

Bode AM, Dong Z. The Amazing and Mighty Ginger. In: Benzie IFF, Wachtel-Galor S, editors. Herbal Medicine: Biomolecular and Clinical Aspects. 2nd edition. Boca Raton (FL): CRC Press/Taylor & Francis; 2011. Chapter 7. Available from: https://www.ncbi.nlm.nih.gov/books/NBK92775/

Serrapeptase

Serrapeptase is an enzyme derived from silkworms. It is especially strong to dissolve scar tissue. The enzyme originated in silkworms, but it is now manufactured in a lab. The silkworm uses this enzyme to dissolve its cocoon. I would be careful to not take too much serrapeptase at one time. I have found it can easily irritate the stomach, because it is so strong. I would take lower doses throughout the day, rather than a large dose at one time.

Serrapeptase is one of the strongest proteolytic enzymes available. I would suggest starting with a lower dose. A common dosage is 40,000 active units.

Serrapeptase can also be called Serratiopeptidase. It can help dissolve excess mucus, sinus congestion, which would relieve cough. Pharmaceuticals used to dissolve mucus can have unwanted side effects. Enzymes are very unlikely to have any side effect. Your body uses its own enzymes to dissolve the mucus in your lungs. It just does not make enough enzymes to keep up with the large amounts that are made during a viral or bacterial infection. Fibrinolytic means to break down fibrin. Mucolytic means to break down mucus.

Research:

Sharma, C., Jha, N. K., Meeran, M., Patil, C. R., Goyal, S. N., & Ojha, S. (2021). Serratiopeptidase, A Serine Protease Anti-Inflammatory, Fibrinolytic, and Mucolytic Drug, Can Be a Useful Adjuvant for Management in COVID-19. *Frontiers in pharmacology*, *12*, 603997. https://doi.org/10.3389/fphar.2021.603997

Nattokinase

Nattokinase is derived from Natto, which is a kind of fermented soybean consumed in Japan. It has been used to relieve blood clots for a long time.

It is interesting that they have already done research on Natto and viruses. It appears that cells treated with natto stopped viruses from infecting cells. In order to prevent a misquote of what the research says, in this case I am providing the abstract.

Research:

Abstract

Natto, a traditional Japanese fermented soybean food, is well known to be nutritious and beneficial for health. In this study, we examined whether natto impairs infection by viruses, such as severe acute respiratory syndrome coronavirus 2 (SARS-CoV-2) as well as bovine herpesvirus 1 (BHV-

1). Interestingly, our results show that both SARS-CoV-2 and BHV-1 treated with a natto extract were fully inhibited infection to the cells. We also found that the glycoprotein D of BHV-1 was shown to be degraded by Western blot analysis and that a recombinant SARS-CoV-2 receptor-binding domain (RBD) was proteolytically degraded when incubated with the natto extract. In addition, RBD protein carrying a point mutation (UK variant N501Y) was also degraded by the natto extract. When the natto extract was heated at 100 °C for 10 min, the ability of both SARS-CoV-2 and BHV-1 to infect to the cells was restored. Consistent with the results of the heat inactivation, a serine protease inhibitor inhibited anti-BHV-1 activity caused by the natto extract. Thus, our findings provide the first evidence that the natto extract contains a protease(s) that inhibits viral infection through the proteolysis of the viral proteins.

Research:

Oba M, Rongduo W, Saito A, Okabayashi T, Yokota T, Yasuoka J, Sato Y, Nishifuji K, Wake H, Nibu Y, Mizutani T. Natto extract, a Japanese fermented soybean food, directly inhibits viral infections including SARS-CoV-2 in vitro. Biochem Biophys Res Commun. 2021 Sep 17;570:21-25. doi: 10.1016/j.bbrc.2021.07.034. Epub 2021 Jul 13. PMID: 34271432; PMCID: PMC8276596.

Lumbrokinase

Lumbrokinase is an enzyme originally derived from earthworms. It is a newer enzyme on the market and appears to be stronger than most enzymes to treat blood clots.

Interestingly, Chinese medicine has used earthworms to treat blood clots, and pain for centuries. It is combined with other herbs, but it is used to break down thick blood, and restore healthy circulation. The name of the herb is Di Long.

Since blood clots are one of the most serious aspects of COVID-19, it appears there is a lot of research being done on using enzymes to thin out the blood naturally and prevent clots.

All of these enzymes can be used to prevent clots from forming in the first place. Taking extra enzymes is one of the best things you can do for your health. According to several sources, Lumbrokinase is 300 times as strong as serrapeptase at dissolving blood clots. Lumbrokinase is 30 times as strong as nattokinase at dissolving clots. I would choose lumbrokinase to dissolve or prevent blood clots, but I would take bromelain, serrapeptase, and nattokinase to treat inflammation.

Research:

Metkar SK, Ghosh S, Girigoswami A, Girigoswami K. The Potential of Serratiopetidase and Lumbrokinase for the Degradation of Prion Peptide 106-126 - an *In Vitro* and *In Silico* Perspective. CNS Neurol Disord Drug Targets. 2019;18(9):723-731. doi: 10.2174/1871527318666191021150002. PMID: 31642793.

Research:

Gioia M, Ciaccio C, Calligari P, De Simone G, Sbardella D, Tundo G, Fasciglione GF, Di Masi A, Di Pierro D, Bocedi A, Ascenzi P, Coletta M. Role of proteolytic enzymes in the COVID-19 infection and promising therapeutic approaches. Biochem Pharmacol. 2020 Dec;182:114225. doi: 10.1016/j.bcp.2020.114225. Epub 2020 Sep 19. PMID: 32956643; PMCID: PMC7501082.

Research:

Wang, Kevin Yueju et al. "Recombinant protein production of earthworm lumbrokinase for potential antithrombotic application." *Evidence-based complementary and alternative medicine : eCAM* vol. 2013 (2013): 783971. doi:10.1155/2013/783971

Another research article I found focuses on blood clots as being possibly the most important aspect of COVID-19. It states that in Wuhan, 90% of hospitalized Covid-19 patients have coagulopathy, which is clotting disorders and thick blood. Preventing blood clots might need to be an important focus in treating this virus. The name of the article is "COVID-19 as a blood clotting disorder masquerading as a respiratory illness."

Research:

Janardhan V, Janardhan V, Kalousek V. COVID-19 as a Blood Clotting Disorder Masquerading as a Respiratory Illness: A Cerebrovascular Perspective and Therapeutic Implications for Stroke Thrombectomy. J Neuroimaging. 2020 Sep;30(5):555-561. doi: 10.1111/jon.12770. Epub 2020 Aug 18. PMID: 32776617; PMCID: PMC7436381.

Enzyme Formulas

In addition to the single enzymes listed above, enzyme formulas are made combining different types of proteases, and other enzymes for a stronger effect. This is what I personally recommend to relieve pain quickly.

One of my favorite products to relieve pain is called Proteolytic Enzymes from Doctor's Best. The dosage is three pills. I believe that most people can get relief from pain without taking pharmaceuticals, if they choose a good product. Another enzyme formula is called FYI Restore, from Garden of Life.

I recently slipped a disc and Proteolytic Enzymes was the only product that allowed me to continue to function. I was barely able to walk. I took two pills an hour for three hours and I was able to walk again. It relieves pain, and dissolves damaged tissue, so the body can heal itself.

Weak and Damaged Veins Can Be Repaired

A common cause of weak veins is high blood sugar levels, and or high insulin. A lot of people have weak blood vessels and do not know it. It appears that COVID-19 damages blood vessels, which can cause circulation and clotting issues.

I tell my patients that if the blood vessels in your legs are weak, the blood vessels in your brain and heart are weak also. I can tell if someone has weak blood vessels, because if they bleed when they get acupuncture, it is often a sign of weak blood vessels. I suggest they take supplements and usually in under seven days, they no longer bleed when they get acupuncture.

Best Vein Supplements

There are two supplements I have used to treat weak veins. The one I currently prefer is Diosmin. This is a bioflavonoid derived from citrus fruit pith. It was originally developed to treat varicose veins, and I find it works very fast, and it is not expensive.

Some companies combine Diosmin with other vein strengthening herbs like horse chestnut.

In my experience, the Diosmin is the most important supplement to use.

I like the Doctor's Best brand. It is called Vein Support. When you look for Diosmin products, you will need to look at the label to ensure how much Diosmin is in it. Each capsule should have at least 400 mg. of Diosmin. Some companies use a lot of fillers. I will not name brands. Of course, adding filler oil to a supplement is not helpful. Herbal capsules should contain 400 to 500 mg. of the active herb.

Another product that can help repair veins is Tru OPC grape seed extract from Nature's Way. This was also developed over 20 years ago to treat varicose veins. Other brands of grape seed extract are not effective, in my experience. OPC is rather expensive, so most companies use filler, and they do not use the exact proanthocyanin that has been shown to be effective.

12

Bronchitis and Pneumonia

This chapter is information for people who have already been diagnosed with either bronchitis or pneumonia. Both these ailments can easily kill you.

I wanted to include this information, including how many people are affected by this, to emphasize why it is so important to treat all colds or flu, or other respiratory infections as quickly as possible. Any type of lung symptoms should send you to your local medical doctor or health center as quickly as possible.

Once you have a diagnosis, you might be prescribed antibiotics. That might help. However, most bronchitis is caused by a virus. The most the antibiotic will do is kill the bacteria building up in the lungs. It will not kill the underlying cause of the infection.

It is estimated that in 2017 there were 49,157 deaths from pneumonia in the US.

Bronchitis is Usually Caused by a Virus

Bronchitis is an inflammation of the bronchial tubes in the lungs. It affects breathing, and can cause intense lung pain and coughing. If bronchitis is not resolved, it can destroy lung function, and it can also be fatal. Most cases of bronchitis are caused by viruses. The antibiotics would help prevent the buildup of bacteria that is probably occurring, but they will not treat the virus. So you are depending on your immune system to do that, with the supplements in this book.

Bronchitis is contagious. So, if you are taking care of someone who has it, it would be advisable to take antiviral supplements yourself, to protect yourself from catching it.

Some cases of bronchitis are caused by bacteria, or fungal infections. It can also be caused by anything that irritates the lungs such as cigarette smoke, dust, and air pollution.

Common symptoms of bronchitis include:

- Sore threat
- Chest tightness, or sensation of fullness
- Wheezing or trouble breathing, especially when lying down
- Fever or chills

- Mucus that is clear, green, or yellow
- Severe coughing, often containing mucus.

Pneumonia is Usually Caused by a Virus

Pneumonia can also be caused by bacteria, viruses, or fungi. About 49,157 deaths were caused by pneumonia in 2017 in the US. Pneumonia is often a result of a viral infection, such as a cold or flu.

Common symptoms of pneumonia include:

- Sore throat
- Fatigue
- Chest pain, possibly stabbing
- Shortness of breath
- Fever
- Mucus that is yellow or green
- Coughing that is severe, and produces mucus.

Symptoms that might be present in pneumonia, but not common in bronchitis are:

- Chills and muscle aches
- Loss of appetite
- Nausea and vomiting, especially in children

- Breathing that is rapid, and shallow. Whereas wheezing is more common in bronchitis
- Mental confusion (possibly caused by reduced oxygen levels)

Pneumonia and bronchitis can be caused by the same infectious pathogens. It is very difficult to tell these diseases apart. It is fortunate that herbs and vitamins that treat viruses often treat bacteria and fungus. They are also often anti-inflammatory.

Bronchitis Patient in His Eighties

I once had a patient in his eighties who was not responding to antibiotics. He had a prescription from his medical doctor for antibiotics, and was told that was all that could be done. He had been sick with bronchitis for over a week, and he could not stop coughing. He seemed to be declining quickly. I knew this was very serious, and it could be deadly at his age.

I gave him the Chinese herb Ban Lan Gen, which is a famous herb called isatis commonly. This resolved his bronchitis in a few days. It is used in Chinese medicine to treat viruses, bacteria, and lung inflammation.

There are many over the counter products that are either single Ban Lan Gen, or combined with other herbs such as dandelion root, which is called taraxacum, or viola, which is a Chinese herb. Each company will have their own formulation. These products are big business in China, so there are many products available. The products often combine the three words and call it Banlangen.

Treat any infection
early and often

Bronchitis and pneumonia can be very deadly for seniors. The following information shows how many people die from lung problems. This table shows the percentage of deaths by age range in the last column.

Flu deaths every year
average 24,000 to
62,000 in the US.

Percentage of flu-related illnesses, medical visits, hospitalizations, and deaths by age group for the 2018-2019 influenza season

	Illnesses	Medical Visits	Hospital-izations	Deaths %
0-4 years	10.2	14.7	5.2	0.8
5-17 years	21.6	24.1	4.3	0.6
18-49 years	33.5	26.7	13.6	7.2
50-64	26.0	24.0	20.0	16.6
65+ years	8.7	10.4	57.0	74.8

Estimated Influenza Disease Burden – United States[1]

Season	**Hospitalizations**		**Deaths**	
	Estimate	**95% UI**	**Estimate**	**95% UI**
2010-2011	**290,000**	(270,000 – 350,000)	37,000	(32,000 – 51,000)
2011-2012	**140,000**	(130,000 – 190,000)	12,000	(11,000 – 23,000)

Estimated Influenza Disease Burden – United States[1]

Season	Hospitalizations		Deaths	
	Estimate	95% UI	Estimate	95% UI
2012-2013	**570,000**	(530,000 – 680,000)	43,000	(37,000 – 57,000)
2013-2014	**350,000**	(320,000 – 390,000)	38,000	(33,000 – 50,000)
2014-2015	**590,000**	(540,000 – 680,000)	51,000	(44,000 – 64,000)
2015-2016	**280,000**	(220,000 – 480,000)	23,000	(17,000 – 35,000)
2016-2017	**500,000**	(380,000 – 860,000)	38,000	(29,000 – 61,000)
2017-2018	**710,000**	(560,000 – 1,100,000)	52,000	(3,000 – 95,500)
2018-2019	**380,000**	(300,000 – 66,000)	28,000	(19,000 – 97,000)

Estimated Influenza Disease Burden – United States[1]

Season	Hospitalizations		Deaths	
	Estimate	95% UI	Estimate	95% UI
2019-2020*	**380,000**	(312,000 – 630,000)	20,000	(18,000 – 80,000)

These tables and references are from Wikipedia, and the CDC.

13

Prevention of Cold and Flu

Your healthy immune system is the most important part of your ability to overcome viral infections. Prevention is the best option. If you take the right supplements, your immune system will be stronger. You will also recover faster, if you do get an infection.

There are many herbs that can improve energy levels and overall resistance to disease. One of the reasons that colds and flu are so dangerous in elderly people is that as we age, we grow weaker. If we are too weak, our bodies do not have the resources to fight off diseases. That is why it is helpful to take tonic herbs. There is a long history of herbal tonics in Chinese medicine. They are antiaging also.

Astragalus

Astragalus can be taken daily to strengthen the immune system, and it also improves digestion and energy levels. It is called Huang Qi in Chinese medicine. Research has shown that it boosts immunity against viruses. A study by Zhang et al, (2018) shows that astragalus polysaccharides can inhibit the replication of avian coronaviruses. There are several immune formulas that contain astragalus and other herbs.

Research:

Zhang P, Liu X, Liu H, Wang W, Liu X, Li X, Wu X. Astragalus polysaccharides inhibit avian infectious bronchitis virus infection by regulating viral replication. Microb Pathog. 2018 Jan;114:124-128. doi: 10.1016/j.micpath.2017.11.026. Epub 2017 Nov 21. PMID: 29170045; PMCID: PMC7126552.

Planetary Herbals makes a product called Full Spectrum Astragalus extract. That would be a good choice for taking the single herb. It would be more effective to take their formula called Astragalus Jade Screen. This is a combination formula that has been used in Chinese medicine for centuries to prevent viral infections and to boost the immune system.

Jade Windscreen

This is a classical Chinese formula that includes the herb astragalus, which is a deep immune tonic. The name Windscreen indicates that it will act to protect you from wind, which is how viruses and allergies are seen in Chinese medicine. Many companies make this formula. The most important herbs are atractylodes, siler root, and astragalus. These should all be herbal extracts.

The Little Boy Who Could Not Play Outside

I had a patient who was about five or six years old. He could not play outside, because he always became sick with allergy symptoms when he did. Since he was so young, I knew that he would respond well to a simple immune tonic, and he did.

After taking Jade Windscreen for less than two months, he could play outside again. His immune system had been strengthened, and pollen and other things outside no longer bothered him. This can often be used to boost the immune system to prevent or treat allergies also.

The Chinese name for Jade Windscreen is Yu Ping Feng San. It contains:

Jade Windscreen

Atractylodes root, Bai Zhu – 40%
Siler root, Fang Feng – 40%
Astragalus, Huang Qi – 20%

Golden Flower Chinese Herbs

This is a simple, yet effective formula to boost the immune system. Many parents in China add raw astragalus root to soups, to improve the immune system and digestion of the whole family. It is a tradition in China to take tonic herbs to boost health.

Jade Windscreen is not enough alone to be used to treat active viral infections. It is used as an immune tonic to strengthen the immune system. It is a gentle, but effective tonic formula.

Jade Windscreen
can be used for:

- Allergies
- Bronchitis
- Cold
- Cough
- Dermatitis
- Flu
- Hives
- Immune system weak
- Meniere's disease
- Nasal discharge

Jade Windscreen Modern Research

Yu Ping Feng San has been researched and shown to prevent viral release and spreading. It also is antibacterial and antiviral. In Chinese medicine terms, it boosts the immune system to prevent invasion. Just about anyone could take this formula to strengthen the immune system over time.

Research:

Du CY, Zheng KY, Bi CW, Dong TT, Lin H, Tsim KW. Yu Ping Feng San, an Ancient Chinese Herbal Decoction, Induces Gene Expression of Anti-viral Proteins and Inhibits Neuraminidase Activity. Phytother Res. 2015 May;29(5):656-61. doi: 10.1002/ptr.5290. Epub 2015 Jan 14. PMID: 25586308.

Cinnamon

Cinnamon is not traditionally used to treat active viral infections in Chinese medicine, so I was very surprised to see a lot of research showing it is effective. According to the Chinese Herbal Materia Medica, by Dan Bensky, "cinnamon has an antibiotic, and very strong inhibitor effect against many gram-positive bacteria, and pathogenic fungi."

I would not personally use it for an active infection, but it would not hurt to take it daily, or to make cinnamon spice tea. It is also used by some people to balance blood sugar.

According to a research report, cinnamon is used in Traditional Persian Medicine. They state that there is an accumulation of inflammatory cells in the lungs that leads to obstruction in asthma, chronic obstructive pulmonary disease, and COVID-19. SARS-Covid-2 infection results in the cilia in the lungs becoming blocked, and mucus is not able to get out.

The cilia are tiny hairs in the lungs that work to push mucus and fluid out of the lungs. If they do not work, the fluid can build up and you cannot breathe. This article states that cinnamon is used in Persian medicine to break down the accumulated mucus, so it can be excreted. It treats lung obstructions.

This article also states that "Inhalation of cinnamon essential oil can improve lung functions and inflammatory conditions."

Research:

Yakhchali M, Taghipour Z, Mirabzadeh Ardakani M, Alizadeh Vaghasloo M, Vazirian M, Sadrai S. Cinnamon and its possible impact on COVID-19: The viewpoint of traditional and conventional medicine. Biomed Pharmacother. 2021 Nov;143:112221. doi: 10.1016/j.biopha.2021.112221. Epub 2021 Sep 21. PMID: 34563952; PMCID: PMC8452493.

Quote "Patient autopsy shows epithelial exfoliation and hyperplasia, mucosa congestion, alveolar damage, exudative inflammation, and thrombosis in infected lungs."

Research

Bian XW; COVID-19 Pathology Team. Autopsy of COVID-19 patients in China. Natl Sci Rev. 2020 Sep;7(9):1414-1418. doi: 10.1093/nsr/nwaa123. Epub 2020 Jun 6. PMID: 34192086; PMCID: PMC7313767.

I would translate that as the lungs are seriously damaged, and mucus has accumulated. The lungs are inflamed, and contain blood clots.

There are two commonly used types of cinnamon. Cinnamon cassia, and verum. Cinnamon verum would be translated as true cinnamon. If you would like to use this herb, Frontier Co-op makes a Ceylon cinnamon, which is supposed to be true cinnamon. It has a sweeter and milder flavor than cinnamon cassia. Several companies also have encapsulated cinnamon. It is easy to take too much cinnamon. If you do this, it will dry out your throat.

There are many herbs that treat mucus accumulation. In Chinese medicine pinellia is used, in combination with other herbs in formulas. However, the underlying virus or bacteria that is causing the infection must be the focus.

Aged Garlic

Garlic is a great supplement to take daily to prevent viral infections. I would not use this to treat an active infection, but it might prevent you from getting one.

You can add garlic to your food, but a good supplement option is Kyolic aged garlic. It is made in Japan and it is aged for two years.

Some supplement companies claim their garlic has more allicin than others, which they say makes it more effective. Allicin is a volatile compound, and it is unlikely to be active in any product by the time it even hits the store.

There are several types of Kyolic formulas. Most of them have added whey protein. This is a common food allergen, and I do not recommend it. I take Kyolic Reserve, it does not have fillers. The dosage is one capsule a day. Although if I were exposed to the virus daily, I would probably take one capsule with each meal. Garlic is also an effective antifungal. It treats Candida and other fungi.

Research:

Pandey, R.K., Pandey, R.K., Shukla, S.S. *et al.* A review on corona virus and treatment approaches with *Allium sativam*. *Futur J Pharm Sci* **7**, 159 (2021). https://doi.org/10.1186/s43094-021-00310-7

Vitamins

In addition to herbs, taking a good multivitamin daily, extra zinc, and adequate vitamin D are important. In order to have a healthy immune system, it needs the raw material to make the immune cells. In my experience, some brands in big box discount stores are not the same quality as those brands sold in health food stores. They are sometimes synthetically derived, and might not be absorbed as well.

Vitamin D

Vitamin D has anti-viral, anti-inflammatory, and immune enhancing actions in the lungs. Vitamin D deficiency is associated with greater COVID-19 disease severity, and vitamin D deficiency is more prevalent among severe cases compared to mild cases.

Research:

Pereira M, Dantas Damascena A, Galvão Azevedo LM, de Almeida Oliveira T, da Mota Santana J. Vitamin D deficiency aggravates COVID-19: systematic review and meta-analysis. Crit Rev Food Sci Nutr. 2020 Nov 4:1-9. doi: 10.1080/10408398.2020.1841090. Epub ahead of print. Update in: Crit Rev Food Sci Nutr. 2021 Aug 12;:1-6. PMID: 33146028.

In order to know your vitamin D levels, you would need to do a blood test. I have not heard of anyone having a reaction to vitamin D supplements at any dosage. I personally take 5,000 mg capsules.

Zinc

Zinc lozenges have been popular for many years to treat colds and flu. Since viruses enter your body through your nose and throat, if zinc is sufficient there, the virus will have a harder time getting to your lungs.

Many people are very deficient in zinc, which puts them at risk of getting more serious viral infections.

I will use a direct quote from a research article.

"As zinc is essential to preserve natural tissue barriers such as the respiratory epithelium, preventing pathogen entry, for a balanced function of the immune system and the redox system, zinc deficiency can probably be added to the factors predisposing individuals to infection and detrimental progression of COVID-19. Finally, due to its direct antiviral properties, it can be assumed that zinc administration is beneficial for most of the population, especially those with suboptimal zinc status."

Research:

Wessels I, Rolles B, Rink L. The Potential Impact of Zinc Supplementation on COVID-19 Pathogenesis. Front Immunol. 2020 Jul 10;11:1712. doi: 10.3389/fimmu.2020.01712. PMID: 32754164; PMCID: PMC7365891.

There are many types of zinc. If I am not sure which type is best, I will look at a brand I trust. They will usually choose the most effective type according to research. Life Extension makes a zinc supplement, it is called Zinc Caps. It has zinc monomethionine, and zinc citrate.

Jarrow makes a product called Zinc Balance. It has one mg. of copper in it. Zinc and copper oppose each other and taking too much of one of these can cause a deficiency in the other one.

I trust both of these products and have used many types of zinc, and cannot tell the difference between them.

Vitamin Deficiencies in COVID-19 Patients

If you take a good daily multivitamin, I personally like Garden of Life Raw vitamins, you will get enough selenium.

According to one research study, 76% of COVID-19 patients were vitamin D deficient, and 42% were selenium deficient.

"In this study, vitamin D and selenium deficiencies were the most prevalent. Additionally, almost all COVID-19 patients with respiratory distress were classified as nutrient-deficient. It is unclear whether individual nutrient deficiencies affected immunity or whether the nutrient deficiency simply led to a decline in the patient's overall condition. However, as it is becoming increasingly clear that hyper-inflammation is a major factor in the course of progression to severe

COVID-19, vitamin D and selenium deficiencies should be highlighted."

Research:

Im, Jae Hyoung et al. "Nutritional status of patients with COVID-19." *International journal of infectious diseases : IJID : official publication of the International Society for Infectious Diseases* vol. 100 (2020): 390-393. doi:10.1016/j.ijid.2020.08.018

From this last quote, you can see that an insurance policy to protect yourself would include a good daily multivitamin, even one pill a day will be very helpful, and vitamin D.

More Prevention Herbs

In addition to the herbs and vitamins in this chapter, please read the cordyceps and curcumin chapters. Both of those herbs can be taken regularly, and both of them have many immune system benefits.

Since herbs are so safe, if I felt I were in danger of getting a serious viral infection, I would not hesitate to take the Chinese formulas, or anything else listed in this book for as long as I felt the need.

14

Cold and Flu Recovery, Long Term Symptoms

Having a viral infection weakens the body. If you cough a lot, your lungs are often weakened also. It is not uncommon for someone to become so worn down by having a virus that they do not seem to ever get over it. Lasting fatigue and a light cough usually mean you either still have an infection, or your body has been weakened and has not recovered.

Boost the Lung Formula

Sometimes people suffer from a weak cough after they recover from a cold, flu, or other viral infection.

There are several options to treat this. One of them is the herbal formula, Bu Fei Tang. This name is translated as Tonify the Lungs Decoction. It contains herbs that strengthen the lungs and stop coughing.

Cordyceps is also a good lung tonic herb. It strengthens the lung energy, as well as the kidneys. Jade Windscreen, explained in the chapter on preventing viral infections, can also be used to help the lungs recover.

Bu Fei Huo Xue – Modern Research

COVID-19 is different from most viruses in that it damages the organs. This can occur with few or no other symptoms. Chinese herbs are being used in China to restore organs damaged by this virus.

Please consult your local acupuncturist for help with this. Each person will have different symptoms that need to be addressed.

The herbal formula being used in China is comprised of:

Astragalus – you know this as an immune tonic herb.

Red peony – this herb is used to cool inflammation and relieve stagnant blood. When you are sick, your blood can get thick, which makes it harder to heal.

Psoralen – This is called Bu Gu Zhi, it is a kidney yang tonic, so it boosts the kidney energy, which is a fast way to boost energy levels to overcome a long illness. This herb strengthens the kidneys, and treats wheezing caused by weak kidneys.

This research article stated that "63% of COVID-19 patients had observable lung damage on

CT scans after being released from the hospital. The formula Bu Fei Huo Xue has been used clinically to prevent and treat pulmonary heart diseases, with Qi deficiency and blood stasis." That means that the person has very low energy levels, and thick blood, and is not recovering from Covid due to this weakness.

The article also states that Psoralen strengthens the heart, and aids in the expansion of the coronary arteries, to promote the increase of blood flow. Using these three herbs together can improve lung function, microcirculation, anti-infection, anti-endotoxin, immunity, resistance to hypoxia, stress, and protect the heart, lung, liver, and kidney functions."

This formula is one of dozens, if not *hundreds* of Chinese herbal formulas that can help people overcome the side effects of a viral or bacterial infection. I have included this information so you know there is hope. So many people get sick and are not able to overcome it. Their body is very worn down it will be hard to fully recover without help.

If I were not an acupuncturist, I would take curcumin or ginger root to thin the blood, and astragalus, and other herbs mentioned in this chapter to improve energy levels. Please read the chapter on blood clot prevention. We all need to consider how to keep our blood circulating as it is supposed to.

I would not try to take this formula on my own, and I would seek the advice of a professional herbalist to get over my symptoms more quickly. No matter how you feel, there is always a way to heal if you get the proper help.

The people who took part in this study had COVID-19, and had not fully recovered. They had a TCM diagnosis of Lung and Spleen Qi deficiency. This means their lungs and digestion were weak. Research:

Chen Y, He W, Lu W, Xing Y, Bai J, Yu H, Zhou J, Liang J, Chen J, Hou C, Zhong B, Wang T, Feng H, Chen X, Wang T, Yang K, Zhang N, Zhong N, Liu C, Wang J. Bufei huoxue capsules in the management of convalescent COVID-19 infection: study protocol for a multicenter, double-blind, and randomized controlled trial. Pulm Circ. 2021 Aug 3;11(3):20458940211032125. doi: 10.1177/20458940211032125. PMID: 34394913; PMCID: PMC8351033.

15

Viruses Are Everywhere - Incurable, or Not?

How many "incurable" diseases are actually caused by infections? One of the reasons I am including this chapter is because so many people have what they believe to be hopeless diseases. They have been told their disease is incurable. Nothing can be done. Their disease is progressive, they will continue to get worse over time, and there is no hope. I don't agree with that. If in doubt, treat it as a virus, and see if it gets better.

Viruses are a major cause of disease. Colds, flu, and COVID-19 are just the most commonly discussed.

If you have a disease, there is always a cause for the disease. Diseases do not just pop up because you have it in your DNA.

Most people do not think about how many different types of viruses there are, and how many diseases they can cause. In addition to all of these known viruses, and the known diseases they cause, there is a lot of research indicating that diseases such as multiple sclerosis, ALS or Lou Gehrig's disease, and even Alzheimer's are either caused by a virus, multiple viruses, bacteria, fungus, or a combination of all of these.

Once you are infected with a pathogen, it is easy to contract another one. There is a lot of research confirming this. Treating viruses with natural medicine is easy. Even if you needed to take supplements every day the rest of your life to stay healthy, it is worth it.

Amyotrophic Lateral Sclerosis (ALS)

Stephen Hawking was a famous physicist who had ALS. This disease is also called Lou Gehrig's disease. ALS is a progressive and considered incurable nerve disease that can cause paralysis. Is this like polio? Polio is caused by a virus, and it can lead to paralysis.

Research has been done that indicates the possibility that this disease is caused by a virus. HERV, which is human endogenous retroviral virus.

Research excerpt:

> "postmortem brain tissue from a number of patients with a classical ALS has revealed significantly increased expression of HERV-K, compared to controls. These findings suggest that endogenous retroviral elements are involved in the pathophysiology of ALS, but there is no evidence that they are the primary cause of the syndrome."

Research:

> Alfahad T, Nath A. Retroviruses and amyotrophic lateral sclerosis. Antiviral Res. 2013 Aug;99(2):180-7. doi: 10.1016/j.antiviral.2013.05.006. Epub 2013 May 23. PMID: 23707220; PMCID: PMC3723705.

Another research article tested the theory that the type of fat consumed might be a factor in ALS. They used extra virgin olive oil for one group of mice, and a standard diet for the other group. They concluded that mice fed extra virgin olive oil "showed a significant higher survival and better motor performance than control mice." The mice on extra virgin olive oil showed better motor performance, and larger muscle fiber area.

As you already know, olive leaf extract is a powerful antiviral. The same compounds in the leaf extract are also present in the oil, only in smaller amounts.

Research:

> Oliván S, Martínez-Beamonte R, Calvo AC, Surra JC, Manzano R, Arnal C, Osta R, Osada J. Extra virgin olive oil intake delays the development of amyotrophic lateral sclerosis associated with reduced reticulum stress and autophagy in muscle of SOD1G93A mice. J Nutr Biochem. 2014

Aug;25(8):885-92. doi: 10.1016/j.jnutbio.2014.04.005. Epub 2014 May 2. PMID: 24917047.

A definition of ALS, quoted directly from www.als.org.

> ALS, or amyotrophic lateral sclerosis, is a progressive neurodegenerative disease that affects nerve cells in the brain and the spinal cord. A-myo-trophic comes from the Greek language. "A" means no. "Myo" refers to muscle, and "Trophic" means nourishment – "No muscle nourishment." When a muscle has no nourishment, it "atrophies" or wastes away. "Lateral" identifies the areas in a person's spinal cord where portions of the nerve cells that signal and control the muscles are located. As this area degenerates, it leads to scarring or hardening ("sclerosis") in the region.
>
> From www.als.org

If this disease is caused by a virus, or bacteria, it is worth a try to treat it with the supplements in this book.

Since this disease is progressive, once the muscles are flaccid, you will need to get physical therapy to activate them again. Acupuncture would also help to restore nerve function.

At one time it was believed that nerves do not regenerate, they also believed the brain was not able to form new brain cells. They now know this is not the case. Our bodies heal and regenerate all the time.

I am not saying that I consider this as a cause of, or cure for ALS, I just think we should keep our minds open and try many things. There has to be a cause for the disease. What caused it? You should ask that over and over until you figure it out. Do not accept a bad prognosis.

If I knew someone with ALS, or any neurological disease, whether it was caused by a brain problem, or a nerve problem, I would treat viruses, bacteria, and Candida, and take high doses of vitamin C. I think most people would benefit from this regimen.

Enteroviruses and ALS

I had to include one more ALS study. Enteroviruses are a type of virus. You are more familiar with rhinoviruses, because they cause the common cold and flu. You are also familiar with coronaviruses. But enteroviruses are in the same family as poliovirus, coxsackievirus, and echovirus. Poliovirus causes polio, which can cause paralysis. These viruses are particularly associated with the central nervous system.

According to one research report, "since the successful campaign of the poliovirus vaccination, neurological diseases caused by non-polio enteroviruses have been increasingly reported."

Let that sink in.

"Acute flaccid paralysis was frequently observed among patients with enterovirus-A71, echovirus, and coxsackievirus infection."

"Viral infection has long been suspected as an environmental risk factor and/or a causative pathogen for ALS."

Research:

Xue YC, Feuer R, Cashman N, Luo H. Enteroviral Infection: The Forgotten Link to Amyotrophic Lateral Sclerosis? Front Mol Neurosci. 2018 Mar 12;11:63. doi: 10.3389/fnmol.2018.00063. PMID: 29593492; PMCID: PMC5857577.

No Incurable Illnesses

Please do not accept any illness as being incurable. In 1995, before I started acupuncture school, I developed neuritis and thoracic outlet syndrome. I had the sensation of needles stabbing my arms all day. I was written off by medical doctors as being incurable. I was in constant pain.

Under no circumstances was I going to accept the idea that I was incurable, and just learn to live with the pain. It turns out that thoracic outlet syndrome is caused by tight shoulder muscles, putting pressure on the nerves in the arms. This cuts off blood flow, and causes inflamed nerves, and you can also lose control over your hands.

Tight shoulder muscles press on the nerves, and without adequate blood flow, the nerves become inflamed, and misfire. Many diseases, including migraines, are caused by blocked blood flow. This is easy to treat with acupuncture.

Walking around campus with a backpack on was one of the things that helped me the most. The backpack pulled my shoulders back, and stretched the shoulder muscles. I am fine now.

I have included my story, because I want you to refuse to accept any chronic illness as incurable. Just because every doctor you consult says nothing can be done, that does not that mean your ailment is incurable. It just means that particular doctor does not know what to do.

As a result of my own chronic pain, I started studying natural medicine. Then in 1996 I started acupuncture school. As an acupuncturist, I have treated many types of "incurable" diseases.

When my patients first come to my office, they usually think they are incurable, but they will try acupuncture anyway. They are desperate. They do not believe me at first, when I tell them I can help them. They often do not understand why no one suggested they try acupuncture.

Unfortunately, there is competition for patients in medicine. Like it or not, that is the truth. Most medical doctors do not understand or believe in acupuncture. Even if they did, they make a living treating patients with drugs and surgery. I know that sounds cynical, and I'm sorry, but I have to tell the truth. Don't wait for someone to refer you to get acupuncture.

Acupuncture is very inexpensive, especially compared to surgery and expensive testing. The results can be fast, and they are lasting results. The underlying cause of the problem is resolved. You do not need to get acupuncture the rest of your life for the same problem. That is not how it works. A complete resolution is expected.

Just because every doctor you consult says nothing can be done, that does not mean that your ailment is incurable. It just means that particular doctor does not know what to do.

Alzheimer's Disease

Alzheimer's disease is characterized by damaged protein in the brain. It is possible that there are viruses, bacteria, and Candida in the brain causing this damage. There is a lot of research on this.

You can do a search online for: PubMed, Alzheimer's, virus, bacteria, Candida, you will find hundreds of research articles exploring these possible factors.

I found the following information very helpful. It states that herpes simplex has been found in the brains of Alzheimer's patients. Antiviral drugs have also shown improvement:

> "Alzheimer's disease (AD) is characterized by the presence of β-amyloid plaques (Aβ) and neurofibrillary tangles (NFTs) in the brain. The prevalence of the disease is increasing and is expected to reach 141 million cases by 2050. Despite the risk factors associated with the disease, there is no known causative agent for AD. Clinical trials with many drugs have failed over the years, and no therapeutic has been approved for AD.
>
> There is increasing evidence that pathogens are found in the brains of AD patients and controls,

such as human herpes simplex virus-1 (HSV-1). Given the lack of a human model, the route for pathogen entry into the brain remains open for scrutiny and may include entry via a disturbed blood-brain barrier or the olfactory nasal route. Many factors can contribute to the pathogenicity of HSV-1, such as the ability of HSV-1 to remain latent, tau protein phosphorylation, increased accumulation of Aβ *in vivo* and *in vitro*, and repeated cycle of reactivation if immunocompromised. Intriguingly, valacyclovir, a widely used drug for the treatment of HSV-1 and HSV-2 infection, has shown patient improvement in cognition compared to controls in AD clinical studies. We discuss the potential role of HSV-1 in AD pathogenesis and argue for further studies to investigate this relationship."

Research:

Sait A, Angeli C, Doig AJ, Day PJR. Viral Involvement in Alzheimer's Disease. ACS Chem Neurosci. 2021 Apr 7;12(7):1049-1060. doi: 10.1021/acschemneuro.0c00719. Epub 2021 Mar 9. PMID: 33687205; PMCID: PMC8033564.

Is Chronic Fatigue Caused by a Virus?

If you can get viruses under control in your body, you might be surprised that you feel a lot better. Chronic fatigue is also likely caused by or associated with a virus. You don't have to know what type of virus it is. The supplements in this book are broad spectrum.

Many modern diseases are still a mystery to researchers. They cannot isolate one specific causative factor. There is no one, single virus they can say caused the disease.

Type	**Transmission**	**Diseases**
Adenovirus	droplet contact[3] fecal-oral[3] venereal[3] direct eye contact[3]	Gastroenteritis[3] Keratoconjunctivitis[3] Pharyngitis[3] Pharyngoconjunctival Fever[3]
Coxsackievirus	fecal-oral[3][27] respiratory[27] droplet contact[3]	Hand, Foot And Mouth Disease[28] Pleurodynia[27] Aseptic Meningitis[27]

Type	**Transmis-sion**	**Diseases**
		Pericarditis Myocarditis
Cytomegalovirus	vertical transmission[3][29][30] bodily fluids[3]	Infectious Mononucleosis[3] Cytomegalic Inclusion Disease[3] Premature Birth[30] Liver, Lung And Spleen Diseases In The Newborn[30] Small Size At Birth[30] Small Head Size[30] Congenital Seizures In The Newborn[30]
Epstein–Barr virus	saliva[3]	Infectious Mononucleosis[3] Burkitt's Lymphoma[3] Hodgkin's Lymphoma Nasopharyngeal Carcinoma
Hepatitis A virus	fecal-oral[3][31]	Acute Hepatitis[3][31]
Hepatitis B virus	bodily fluids[3]	Acute Hepatitis[3][32]

Type	Transmis-sion	Diseases
	Vertical and sexual[32]	Chronic Hepatitis[32] Hepatic Cirrhosis[32] Hepatocellular Carcinoma[32]
Hepatitis C virus	blood[3] sexual contact[3]	Acute Hepatitis[3][33] Chronic Hepatitis[3] Hepatic Cirrhosis[3] Hepatocellular Carcinoma[3]
Herpes simplex virus, type 1	direct contact[3][29] saliva[3][29]	Herpes Labialis,[3] Cold Sores[3][29] – Can Recur By Latency[3] Gingivostomatitis In Children[3] Tonsillitis & Pharyngitis In Adults[3] Keratoconjunctivitis[3]
Herpes simplex virus, type 2	sexual contact[3][29] vertical transmission[3][29]	Skin Vesicles, Mucosal Ulcers,[29] Oral And/Or Genital[29] Can Be Latent[3] Aseptic Meningitis[3]
HIV	sexual contact[3][34]	Aids[3]

Type	**Transmission**	**Diseases**
	blood[3][34] breast milk[3][34] vertical transmission	
Human coronavirus 229E (HCoV-229E)	droplet contact fomites	Common Cold Pneumonia Bronchiolitis
Human coronavirus NL63 (HCoV-NL63)	droplet contact	Common Cold Rhinitis Bronchitis Bronchiolitis Pneumonia Croup
Human coronavirus OC43 (HCoV-OC43)		Common Cold Pneumonia
Human coronavirus HKU1 (HCoV-HKU1)		Common Cold Pneumonia Bronchiolitis
Human herpesvirus, type 8	Saliva[29] Sexual[29]	Kaposi Sarcoma[3]

Type	Transmission	Diseases
		Multicentric Castleman Disease[3] Primary Effusion Lymphoma[3]
Human papillomavirus	direct contact[3][35] sexual contact[35] vertical transmission	(Common, Flat, Plantar And Anogenital Warts, Laryngeal Papillomas, Epidermodysplasia Verruciformis)[3] Malignancies For Some Species (Cervical Carcinoma,[35] Squamous Cell Carcinomas)[3]
Influenza virus	droplet contact[3]	Influenza[3] (Reye Syndrome)[3]
Measles virus	droplet contact[3][22]	Measles[3][22] Postinfectious Encephalomyelitis[3]
Middle East respiratory syndrome-related coronavirus (MERS-CoV)	close human contact	Middle East Respiratory Syndrome (MERS)
Mumps virus	droplet contact[3][22]	Mumps[3][22]
Parainfluenza virus	droplet contact[3][22]	Croup[3] Pneumonia[3]

Type	Transmission	Diseases
		Bronchiolitis[3] Common Cold[3]
Poliovirus	fecal-oral[3]	Poliomyelitis[3]
Rabies virus	animal bite[3][24] droplet contact[3]	Rabies[3] (Fatal Encephalitis)[24]
Respiratory syncytial virus	droplet contact[3][22] hand to mouth[3]	Bronchiolitis[3] Pneumonia[3] Influenza-Like Syndrome[3] Severe Bronchiolitis With Pneumonia[3]
Rubella virus	Respiratory[36] d roplet contact[3]	Congenital Rubella[3][36] German Measles[3]
Severe acute respiratory syndrome coronavirus (SARS-CoV)	droplet contact	Severe Acute Respiratory Syndrome (SARS)
Severe acute respiratory syndrome coronavirus 2 (SARS-CoV-2)	droplet contact	Coronavirus Disease 2019 (COVID-19)
Varicella-zoster virus	droplet contact[3] direct contact	Chickenpox[29] Herpes Zoster[3]

Type	Transmission	Diseases
		Congenital Varicella Syndrome[29]

16

Shocking Ways Viruses Can Cause Chronic Diseases

The number of diseases that are believed to be caused by viruses, bacteria, or fungus grows by the day. I was surprised to find the following information on Wikipedia. I have been researching autoimmune diseases, and viral diseases for many years, but I did not have enough mainstream confirmation until now.

If you or someone you love has any of the following diseases, and it is not responding to other treatments, you could try the remedies in this book, and see if it improves.

Candida is a fungus that is normally not harmful to us, until it grows out of control. It can also infect the brain, causing a variety of neurological diseases.

Bear in mind that research is ongoing on the cause or causes of many diseases. It is difficult for scientists to isolate viruses in the body. They also do not know about all viruses, so they would not be able to identify them.

I believe most diseases are curable if the underlying cause is treated, and they are caught in time. Toxicity is not included in this list. That is also a common cause of disease in modern times.

Asthma	*Mycoplasma pneumoniae*[4] and *Chlamydia pneumoniae* infections are associated with the onset and symptoms of asthma.[5]
Autoimmune diseases	Autoimmune diseases are associated with *Neoehrlichia mikurensis* infection, and *Borrelia miyamotoi* infection,[1] and HIV,[6] and the bacterium *Mycobacterium tuberculosis*.[7] Autoimmune thyroid disease is associated with Epstein-Barr virus.[8]
Cancer	**Anal cancer** is associated with human papillomaviruses.[9] **Bladder cancer** Schistosoma helminths can cause cancer.[10] **Brain tumor**. Glioblastoma multiforme is associated with cytomegalovirus,[11] BK virus, JC virus, and simian virus 40.[12] **Breast cancer** is associated with mouse mammary tumor virus, Epstein-Barr virus, and human papillomaviruses.[13] **Carcinoid tumors** are associated with enterovirus infections.[14] **Cervical cancer** can be caused by human papillomaviruses.[15][16] **Colorectal cancer** is associated with the bacteria *Helicobacter pylori*, *Streptococcus bovis* and *Fusobacterium nucleatum*,[17] with human

	papillomaviruses,[18] and with the helminth *Schistosoma japonicum*.[19] JC virus may be a risk factor for colorectal cancer.[20] **Gallbladder cancer** is associated with the bacterium *Salmonella* Typhi.[21] **Hodgkin's lymphoma** is associated with Epstein-Barr virus,[22] hepatitis C virus,[23] and HIV.[24] **Kaposi's Sarcoma** can be caused by Kaposi's sarcoma herpesvirus and HIV. **Liver cancer**. Hepatocellular carcinoma can be caused by hepatitis B virus, hepatitis C virus,[25] and by the helminth *Schistosoma japonicum*.[26] **Lung cancer** is associated with the bacterium *Chlamydia pneumoniae*,[27] with human papillomaviruses, and with Merkel cell polyomavirus.[28] **Leukemia**. Adult T-cell leukemia can be caused by human T-cell leukemia virus-1. **Mesothelioma** is associated with simian virus 40,[29] especially in conjunction with asbestos exposure. **Nasopharyngeal carcinoma** can be caused by Epstein-Barr virus. **Non-Hodgkin lymphoma** is associated with HIV and simian virus 40.[30] **Oropharyngeal cancer** can be caused by human papillomaviruses. **Ovarian cancer** is associated with mumps virus. **Pancreatic cancer** is associated with hepatitis B virus and the bacterium *Helicobacter pylori*. **Prostate cancer** is associated with xenotropic murine leukemia virus-

	related virus and BK virus. **Skin neoplasm** is associated with human papillomaviruses. **Squamous cell carcinoma** is associated with human papillomaviruses. **Stomach cancer** is associated with the bacterium *Helicobacter pylori*. **Thyroid cancer** is associated with simian virus 40.
Chronic fatigue syndrome	Chronic fatigue syndrome (also known as myalgic encephalomyelitis) is associated with enteroviruses (such as Coxsackie B virus),[31][32] human herpesvirus 6 variant A,[33] human herpesvirus 7,[34] and parvovirus B19.[35][36] The bacteria *Coxiella burnetii*[37] and *Chlamydia pneumoniae*[38] are known causes of chronic fatigue syndrome (antibiotics can cure these bacterial forms of chronic fatigue syndrome).
Common cold	The common cold is also known as Acute rhinosinusitis (ARS) and is caused by a viral infection.[39] Efforts to develop vaccines are ongoing.[2]
Crohn's disease	One study found ileocecal Crohn's disease is associated with viral species from the enterovirus genus (but note that all the study cohort with ileocecal Crohn's disease had disease-associated mutations in either their NOD2 or ATG16L1 genes).[40] Crohn's disease is associated with *Mycobacterium avium* subspecies *paratuberculosis*.[41] In a murine model, Crohn's disease is

	precipitated by the norovirus CR6 strain,[3][42] but only in combination with a variant of the Crohn's susceptibility gene ATG16L1, and chemical toxic damage to the gut. In other words, in this mouse model, Crohn's is precipitated only when these three causal factors (virus, gene, and toxin) act in combination.
Coronary heart disease	Coronary heart disease is associated with herpes simplex virus 1 and the bacterium *Chlamydia pneumoniae*.[43]
Dementia	Dementia is associated with herpes simplex virus type 1, herpes simplex virus type 2, cytomegalovirus, West Nile virus, bornavirus, and HIV. Dementia is also associated with the helminth *Taenia solium* (pork tapeworm), and with *Borrelia* species bacteria.[44]
Depression	Depression is associated with cytomegalovirus[45] and West Nile virus,[46] and the protozoan parasite Toxoplasma gondii.[47] It is thought that depression may be precipitated by the effect of immune signals (such as pro-inflammatory cytokines) reaching the brain from infections located in the peripheries of the body.[48][49] **Major depressive disorder** is associated with bornavirus,[50] as well as Bartonella[51] and *Borrelia*[44] species bacteria. **Seasonal affective disorder** is associated with Epstein-Barr virus.[52]

Diabetes mellitus type 1	Diabetes mellitus type 1 is associated with viral species from the enterovirus genus,[53][54] specifically ech ovirus 4[55] and Coxsackie B virus (the latter it is thought may infect and destroy the insulin producing beta-cells in the pancreas and also damage these cells via indirect autoimmune mechanisms).[56][57] One study found Coxsackie B1 virus associated with a higher risk of the beta cell autoimmunity that portends type 1 diabetes; though Coxsackie B3 and B6 viruses were found to be associated with a *reduced* risk of such autoimmunity (possibly due to immune cross-protection against Coxsackie B1 virus).[58] In boys, human parechovirus infection has been linked to a subsequent appearance of diabetes-associated autoantibodies.[59]
Diabetes mellitus type 2	Diabetes mellitus type 2 is associated with cytomegalovirus,[60] hepatitis C virus,[61] enteroviruses,[54] Ljungan virus[62]
Dilated cardiomyopa thy	Dilated cardiomyopathy is associated with enteroviruses such as Coxsackie B virus.[63]
Epilepsy	Epilepsy is associated with human herpesvirus 6.[64]
Gonorrhea	Men who have had a gonorrhea infection have a risk of having prostate cancer.[65]
Guillain–Barré syndrome	Guillain–Barré syndrome is associated with the bacterium *Campylobacter jejuni*, and with the

	viruses cytomegalovirus[66] and enteroviru s.[67]
Irritable bowel syndrome	Irritable bowel syndrome (IBS) is associated with the bacteria enteroaggregative *Escherichia coli*[68] and *Mycobacterium avium* subspecies *paratuberculosis*,[69] the protozoan parasite *Giardia lamblia*,[70] and pathogenic strains of the protozoan parasite *Blastocystis hominis*.[71] Irritable bowel syndrome in those with HIV is associated with the protozoan *Dientamoeba fragilis*.[72]
Low back pain	Lower back pain is associated with a spinal disc infection with anaerobic bacteria, especially the bacterium *Cutibacterium acnes*.[73][74]
Lupus	Lupus is associated with the viruses parvovirus B19,[75] Epstein-Barr virus,[76] and cytomegalovirus.[77]
Lyme disease	Lyme disease is associated with infection by *Borrelia miyamotoi*, and *Rickettsia* species.[1]
Metabolic syndrome	Metabolic syndrome is associated with the bacteria *Chlamydia pneumoniae*[78] and *Helicobacter pylori*, as well as the viruses cytomegalovirus and herpes simplex virus 1.[79]
Multiple sclerosis	Multiple sclerosis, a demyelinating disease, is associated with Epstein-Barr virus[80] (and strongly associated with

	certain genetic variants of this virus),[81] human herpesvirus 6,[82] varicella zoster virus,[83] and the bacterium *Chlamydia pneumoniae*.[84]
Myocardial infarction	Myocardial infarction (heart attack) is associated with *Chlamydia pneumoniae*,[85] cytomegalovirus[86] and Co xsackie B virus (an enterovirus).[87] (Coxsackie B virus is also associated with sudden unexpected death due to myocarditis).[88]
Obesity	Obesity is associated with adenovirus 36, which is found in 30% of obese people, but only in 11% of non-obese people.[89][90] It has further been demonstrated that animals experimentally infected with adenovirus 36 (or adenovirus 5, or adenovirus 37) will develop increased obesity.[91] Adenovirus 36 induces obesity by infecting fat cells (adipocytes), wherein the expression of the adenovirus E4orf1 gene turns on both the cell's fat producing enzymes and also instigates the generation of new fat cells.[92] Evidence suggests that obesity can be a viral disease, and that the worldwide obesity epidemic that began in the 1980s may be in part due to viral infection.[93][94] Obesity is also associated with higher gut levels of certain Firmicutes bacteria in relation to Bacteroidetes bacteria. Overweight individuals tend have more Firmicutes bacteria (such as *Clostridium*, *Staphylococcus*, *Streptococ cus*, and *Helicobacter pylori*) in their gut,

	whereas normal weight individuals tend have more Bacteroidetes bacteria.[95]
Obsessive–compulsive disorder	Obsessive–compulsive disorder is associated with *Streptococcus*[96] and *Borrelia*[44] speci es bacteria.
Panic disorder	Panic disorder is associated with *Borrelia*[44] and *Bartonella*[51] species bacteria.[51]
Parkinson's disease	Parkinson's disease is associated with influenza A virus,[97] as well as the protozoan parasite *Toxoplasma gondii*.[98]
Psoriasis	Psoriasis is associated with a *Helicobacter pylori* trigger.[99]
Rheumatoid arthritis	Rheumatoid arthritis is associated with parvovirus B19.[75]
Sarcoidosis	Sarcoidosis is associated with Mycobacteria[100] species and the bacterium *Helicobacter pylori*[101]
Schizophren-ia	Schizophrenia is associated with bornavirus,[50] the bacterium *Chlamydia trachomatis*,[102] as well as *Borrelia* species bacteria.[44] Schizophrenia is also linked to neonatal infection with Coxsackie B virus (an enterovirus), which one study found carries an increased risk of adult onset schizophrenia.[103] Prenatal exposure to influenza virus in the first trimester of pregnancy increases the risk of schizophrenia by 7-fold.[104]

Severe acute respiratory syndrome	Severe acute respiratory syndrome is a viral disease. Efforts to develop a vaccine are ongoing.[2]
Stroke	Stroke is associated with the bacteria *Chlamydia pneumoniae*,[105] *Helicobacter pylori*,[106] *Mycobacterium tuberculosis*,[107] and *Mycoplasma pneumoniae*,[108] as well as the virus varicella zoster virus[109] and *Histoplasma* species fungi.[110]
Thromboangiitis obliterans	Thromboangiitis obliterans is associated with *Rickettsia* species bacteria.[111]
Tourette syndrome	Tourette syndrome is associated with *Streptococcus* species bacteria.[112] Aggravating or contributory microbes in Tourette's may include the bacteria *Mycoplasma pneumoniae*,[113] *Chlamydia pneumoniae*, *Chlamydia trachomatis*, and the protozoan parasite *Toxoplasma gondii*.[114]
Vasculitis	Vasculitis is associated with HIV, parvovirus B19,[75] and hepatitis B virus. The hepatitis C virus is an established cause of vasculitis.

Index

References

Chinese Herbal Medicine Materia Medica, by Dan Bensky

The Infection Game, by Dr. Sarah Myhill, and Craig Robinson

Primal Panacea, by Thomas E. Levy, MD, JD www.PeakEnergy.com.

The website www.DrJakeFratkin.com for the most current research on Chinese herbal medicine in the treatment of modern viral outbreaks.

Clinical Guide to Commonly Used Chinese Herbal Formulas, John Scott, DOM, Lorena Monda, DOM, John Heuertz, DOM (Catalog for Golden Flower Chinese Herbs)

Dissolving Illusions, Disease, Vaccines, and the Forgotten History by Suzanne Humphries, MD, Roman Bystrianyk.

Other Books by Deborah Bleecker

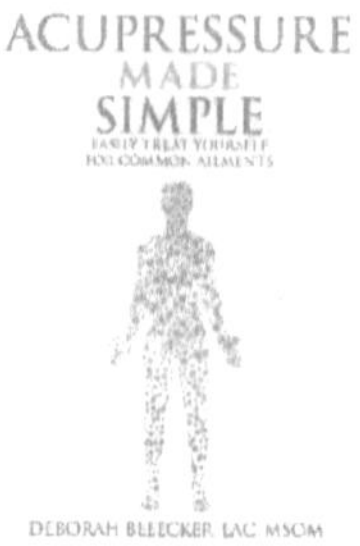

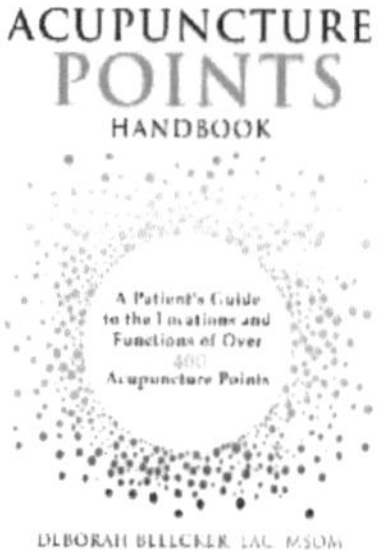

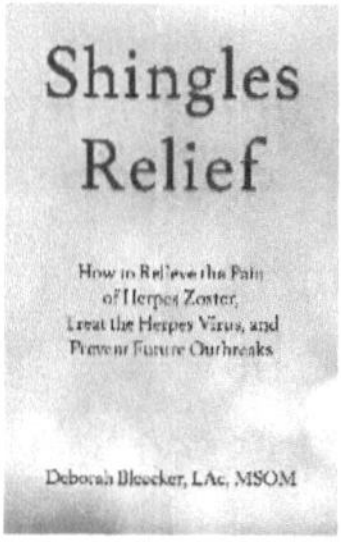

Also, from This Publisher

Dallas Designs Notebooks, available only on Amazon. Dozens of designs. Animals, flowers, and abstract notebook designs. Three different sizes.

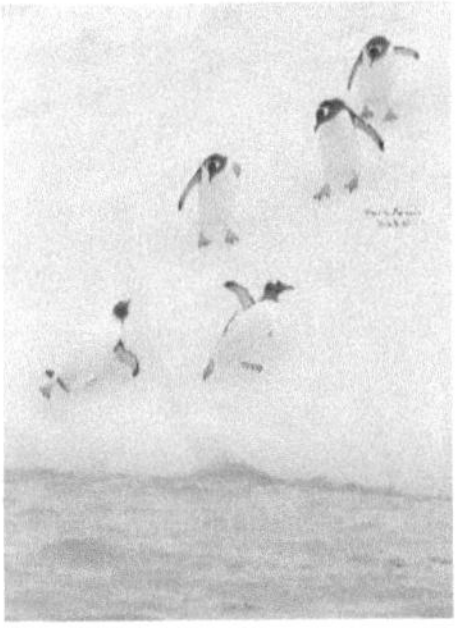
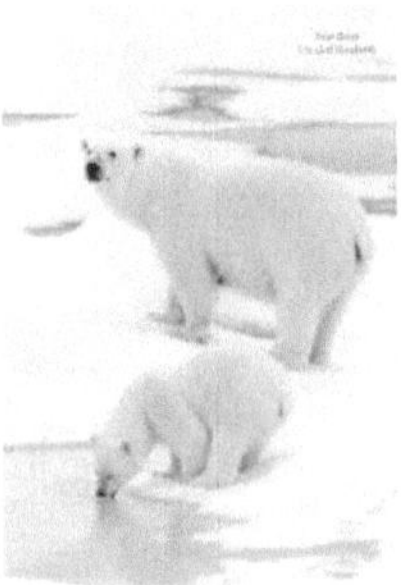
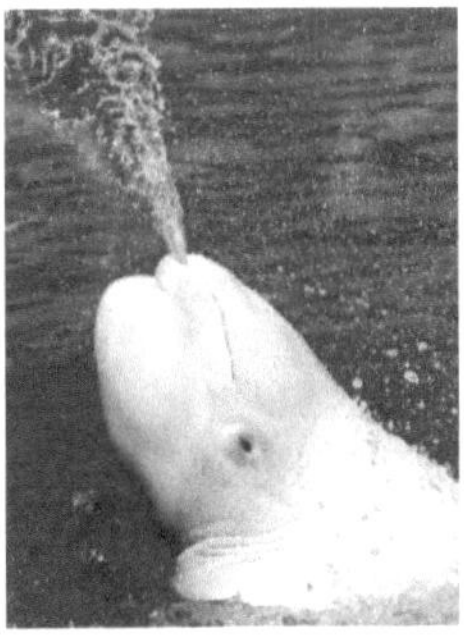
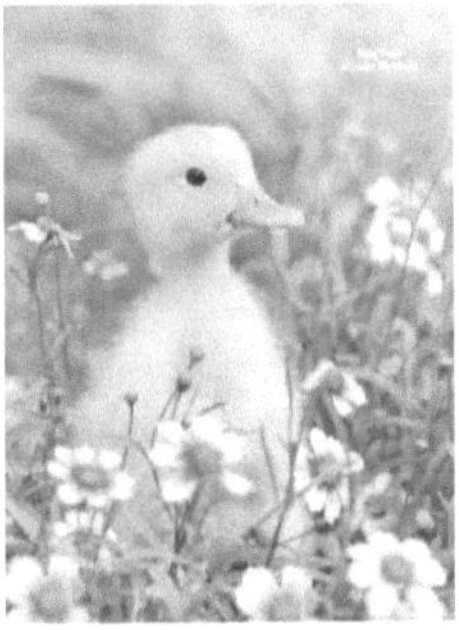
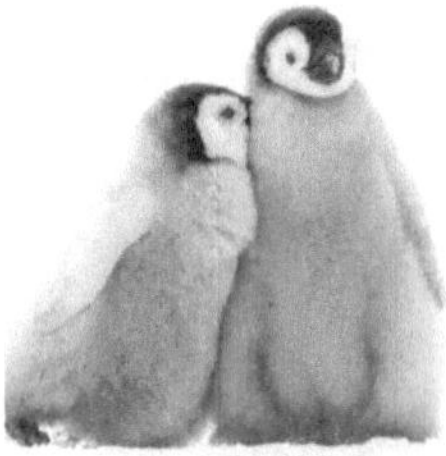
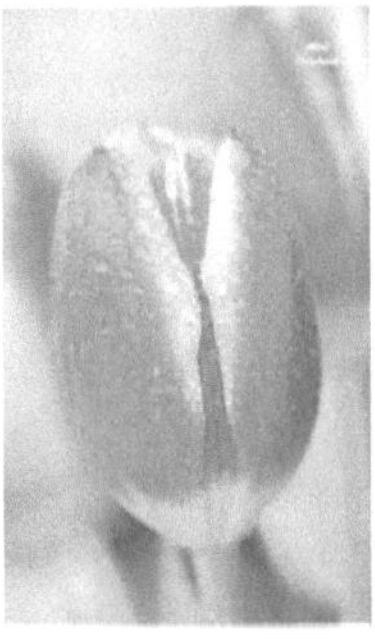
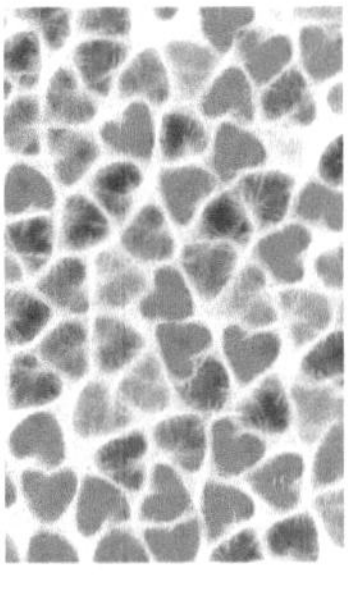

Made in United States
Troutdale, OR
09/05/2026

54097160R00116